Jan Clark was born in Sussex and now lives in Bristol where she works as a counsellor in private practice. She co-founded the Hysterectomy Support Network (Avon) in 1990, is married to a retired chiropractor and has two grown-up children and a granddaughter.

WITHDRAWN

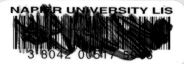

Hysterectomy
and the
Alternatives

*How to ask the right questions
and explore other options*

Jan Clark

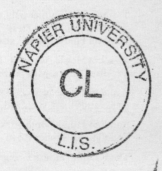

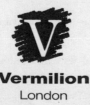

Vermilion
London

This book is dedicated to all the women
who contributed so much to my research between the
years 1990–2000 and made this book possible.

Thank you.

1 3 5 7 9 10 8 6 4 2

Text © Jan Clark 2000
Illustrations © Random House Group Ltd 2000

Jan Clark has asserted her right to be identified as the author of this work
under the Copyright, Designs and Patents Act 1988.

First published in the United Kingdom in 1993 by Virago Press

This new edition first published in the United Kingdom in 2000 by Vermilion,
an imprint of Ebury Press
Random House, 20 Vauxhall Bridge Road, London SW1V 2SA

Random House Australia (Pty) Limited
20 Alfred Street, Milsons Point, Sydney, New South Wales 2061, Australia

Random House New Zealand Limited
18 Poland Road, Glenfield, Auckland 10, New Zealand

Random House South Africa (Pty) Limited
Endulini, 5A Jubilee Road, Parktown 2193, South Africa

The Random House Group Limited Reg. No. 954009

www.randomhouse.co.uk

A CIP catalogue record for this book is available from the British Library.

ISBN 0 09 185612 4

Printed and bound at Cox and Wyman, Reading, Berks

Papers used by Vermilion are natural, recyclable products made from
wood grown in sustainable forests.

Contents

Acknowledgements

My thanks go to the following who contributed their professional expertise, practical assistance and kindness:

Professor Peter Braude FRCOG, Guy's and St Thomas NHS Trust, London. **Wendy Landow,** *Director of Research* SCVIR, (USA). **Dr Woodruff Walker,** *Consultant Radiologist*, Royal Surrey County Hospital. **Dr James Browning,** *Director*, Gynecare, Edinburgh. **Dr David E Parkin,** *Consultant Gynaecologist*, Aberdeen Royal Infirmary. **Mr Nicholas Sharp,** *Consultant Gynaecologist*, Royal United Hospital, Bath. **Dr John Reidy,** *Consultant Radiologist*, Guy's & St Thomas NHS Trust, London. **Dr Phillippa Cheetham,** Oxford. **Mary Grinsted,** *Statistical Officer*, Department of Health, London. **Lindsay Appleton.**

My thanks as well to my husband for his continuing emotional and practical support.

Preface

Hysterectomy is the most common surgical operation performed by gynaecologists; some 80,000 being performed in the UK annually and around half a million performed annually in the USA. It is thus not surprising that the ubiquity of this operation is being questioned and less invasive alternatives being sought, both by women and their gynaecologists.

Many women wish to explore alternatives to surgery and therefore investigate other measures that might be effective. Those who have little alternative and require the hysterectomy for sound medical reasons, often find it difficult to obtain clear guidance on what they might expect of the operation and how they might prepare themselves for it, both before and after surgery.

Jan Clark has provided this helpful and informative book to answer these very questions. It is a clear and logical account of the medical alternatives to hysterectomy and offers helpful advice, not found easily in either medical or non-medical textbooks, about the surgery itself, preparing for it and dealing with its aftermath, including the need for Hormone Replacement Therapy when appropriate. Alternative measures such as acupuncture, medical herbalism and homoeopathy are all given a fair hearing. This account will be useful for those who wish to try these measures when the need for surgery is not clear.

Women around the country will be grateful for this book, as with increasing demands both on patients and doctors, each of whom lead increasingly busy lives, the time for discussion, information giving, synthesis and decision making is often limited. *Hysterectomy and the Alternatives* provides the opportunity for each woman to explore the issues herself, to develop the understanding needed to ask sensible and relevant questions, and where these are not forthcoming, to be able to make informed choices herself. It is an important book.

Professor Peter Braude
Consultant Obstetrician & Gynaecologist
Head of the Division of Women's and Children's Health at the
Guy's, King's and St Thomas' School of Medicine
October 2000

Foreword

My friend, Lorraine, had a hysterectomy five years ago.

'Nothing to it!' she exclaimed when she heard I was about to have one. 'Don't know what all the fuss is about! I went dancing two weeks after the operation – I've never looked back!'

Mine was on 11 August 1988, one of an estimated 80,000 in the UK that year. I was frightened of it, partly because I am not the ideal patient, someone who can relax and allow it all to happen. I am also terrified of anaesthesia and, having had two children by Caesarean section, didn't relish the idea of a third abdominal incision.

All these fears swirled around in my mind, as I listened to comments endorsing Lorraine's words – 'You'll feel a new woman! . . . so fit and energetic . . . fantastic!' But, I protested, I didn't feel ill and there was nothing to show for what was going on inside me, no outward signs of distress. It was difficult to imagine an 'improved me' afterwards.

At that time I held a temporary administrative post within Bristol RELATE. Every day, at least one counsellor or member of staff who had a few free minutes came to ask how I was and encouraged me to talk about my anxieties. I owe them all an enormous debt of gratitude.

My doctor had explained it to me in more detail and answered my questions clearly and reassuringly. Yet strangely enough – though I didn't think so at the time – he didn't say 'I suggest you buy such and such a book, it's very helpful', or even offer a leaflet. Quite why I never went to the library and looked for information is something I will never know.

So I went into hospital and returned two weeks later. Most of the following six weeks was taken up with treating an infected abdominal incision and struggling to become mobile again, for I am a woman with a physical disability. I had never felt so tired and it was during this weak-as-a-kitten stage that

I began to ask questions during occasional bouts of lucid thinking: Were there more women having hysterectomies than, say, five years ago? If so, why? How did women without partners and/or families manage? In my innocence I'd always associated hysterectomy with the menopause, yet there had been a couple of very young women in the ward . . .

It took just over a year before I felt really fit again. Later, in the course of writing this book when hundreds of women wrote to me about this event in their lives, I realised that Lorraine's and my experiences of the same operation were the opposite ends of the spectrum, that the average experience of it is somewhere in the middle.

When I wrote my book in 1993, I stated that in the past ten years the annual hysterectomy rate in NHS Hospitals in the UK had fluctuated but overall the numbers were rising. They still continue to hover around 80,000 but there has been a steady increase in the use of alternative treatments, such as endometrial ablation, which have increased from 11,000 to 16,000 in the corresponding time. And these figures take no account of women who are using complementary therapy.

This is good news. It means women now have real choice, particularly those suffering from menstrual disorders for which most hysterectomies are performed. Does it matter if the alternatives are not explored? I believe it does, partly because hysterectomy may not always be the right answer and partly because all surgery carries some risk, especially major surgery. To put oneself at risk without at least first exploring other options seems to me to be short-sighted.

Doctors still need to be made aware there are alternatives to major surgery – too often it is patients who draw attention to them, with articles extracted from newspapers and magazines. There is at least growing evidence of GPs and complementary therapists sharing medical practices which can only be to the benefit of patients.

This book is for *you* – the woman who may be considering whether or not to have a hysterectomy. I hope you will share it with someone close to you.

Jan Clark
October 2000

Chapter One

Knowing What to Expect

Most people are in awe of specialists and don't know what to ask. Rosemary (Mid-Glamorgan)

As far as information being available – it wasn't. Locally I couldn't find anything to help me. The consultant just patted my head and told me not to be a silly girl, that there was nothing to the operation. Sue (Dorset)

These two extracts from letters sent to me by women who had experienced hysterectomy may have struck a chord with you.

Perhaps you have an appointment with the specialist next week and you are anxious about talking to a total stranger in unfamiliar surroundings: you know that something has to be done, you can't take any more of the pain, but you are frightened there is something seriously wrong and you were shocked when your sister mentioned the word hysterectomy. What does that mean? and who will look after the children? You recall fragments of anxious conversations when your mother or grandmother went into hospital and vaguely remember reading an article about hysterectomy in a magazine. Your best friend is sympathetic but cannot really help. It all seems totally overwhelming.

Or maybe you have already seen the specialist but felt confused at the end of the brief consultation with a white-coated figure of medical authority. Seeing the specialist as 'the expert', you were frightened to disagree when told your womb should be removed. But you are not sure if it really is the right answer to your problems, and you are puzzled that the date of the operation was fixed at the consultation as you thought there was a waiting list. You feel annoyed with yourself because you cannot remember exactly what was said about your ovaries, yet it seemed clear at the time of the consultation.

If you identify with some of these feelings, you are not alone. You share them with thousands of women concerned

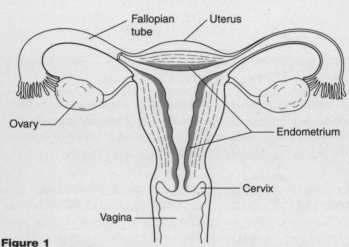

Figure 1

At the centre of your sexual and reproductive organs is your **uterus** (womb). This is a thickly walled and muscular organ, about 3 inches long and 2 inches wide, which looks like an upside-down pear. The darkest shaded area in the illustration is the **endometrium**, a soft pink layer of tissue which is rich in blood vessels, and this lines the whole of the uterine cavity. Most of it decays and is shed during your periods.

Each end of the top of the uterus opens into two tubes – your **Fallopian** tubes. You can see how they curl forwards, their endings like the fronds of a sea anemone, and they move closer to your **ovaries** when the release of an egg is imminent.

These organs are attached to ligaments, or bands of strong tissue. All your pelvic organs are flexible, and not simply fixed in one place.

At the lower end of your uterus is your **cervix** which opens into your **vagina**: there are folds of layered tissue surrounding your vagina and these spread out and expand in response to your thoughts, feelings and needs, which might be fingers, a tampon, a penis, or to relax and let a baby slither out at birth.

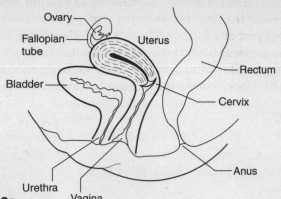

Figure 2a

This shows how your uterus is situated in relation to your **bladder** (which stores your urine until it is released via your **urethra**) and your **rectum** (or back passage) down which waste matter is expelled through your **anus**.

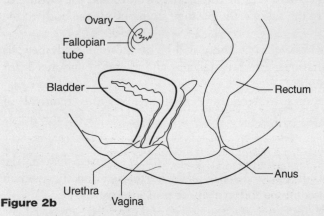

Figure 2b

Here are the same organs once your uterus has been surgically removed. It looks as though there will be a large internal empty space, but the coils of your intestine unwind sufficiently to fill it.

about possible hysterectomy. It is quite normal if you cannot think straight at the moment, cannot concentrate on one aspect of potential disruption to your life without other worrying thoughts intruding.

Making sense of your situation and resolving fears and anxieties is possible now that you have chosen to learn as much as you need about hysterectomy, and to consider whether there are alternative solutions to your particular gynaecological problems. As your understanding of the implications of surgical and non-surgical treatments increases, so confidence and ease of mind will replace much of the present stress. The more you feel you have been involved in the decision as to whether or not you should have a hysterectomy, the more you will feel in control of your life, and the less likely you are to regret the decision you make.

What is a Hysterectomy?

The word hysterectomy is a combination of two Greek words – *hyster* (uterus) and *ektome* (to cut out). Hysterectomy means the surgical removal of the uterus (womb) and the closing of the top of the vagina (the passage from outside the body to the uterus).

After hysterectomy there will be no more monthly periods (menstruation), no pregnancies and therefore no need for contraception.

Sometimes hysterectomy also involves the removal of other organs. The different kinds of surgical procedures are as follows:

- *Sub-total hysterectomy:* the uterus is removed, leaving the cervix in place. This is rarely performed and the woman must continue to have smear tests afterwards.
- *Total hysterectomy:* the uterus and cervix are removed.
- *Total hysterectomy with oophorectomy* (removal of one ovary).
- *Total hysterectomy with bilateral oophorectomy* (removal of both ovaries).
- *Total hysterectomy with salpingo-oophorectomy* (removal of the Fallopian tube and ovary on one side).
- *Total hysterectomy with bilateral salpingo-oophorectomy* (removal of both ovaries and both Fallopian tubes).

- *Wertheim's hysterectomy* (also called extended or radical hysterectomy): the uterus, part of the vagina, the Fallopian tubes, usually the ovaries, as well as the lymph glands and fatty tissue in the pelvis are all removed.

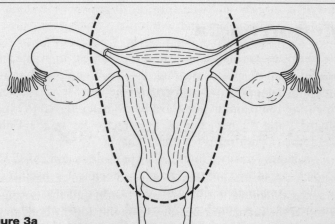

Figure 3a

This shows a **total hysterectomy**: the uterus and cervix are removed with the supporting ligaments. The ovaries and Fallopian tubes remain.

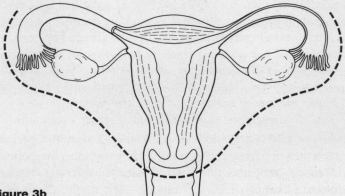

Figure 3b

This shows a **total hysterectomy with bilateral salpingo-oophorectomy**: the uterus, cervix, ovaries and Fallopian tubes are removed.

A woman can be advised to have a hysterectomy for any of the following reasons, some of which can be inter-linked (i.e. co-existing fibroids and PID) :

MENORRHAGIA, FIBROIDS, ENDOMETRIOSIS, PELVIC INFLAMMATORY DISEASE, PROLAPSE, CANCER

Menorrhagia

The term menorrhagia is from the Greek *men* meaning 'month' and *rhegynae* meaning 'to rush out', and it is a complaint of excessive menstrual bleeding. It is the main presenting complaint in one-third of women referred to gynaecologists, and 42 per cent of hysterectomies in the United Kingdom are performed for menorrhagia.

A woman's fertility, and thus her periods, is controlled by a complex set of hormones. These are chemical substances in the bloodstream that fluctuate during her menstrual cycle. This begins in a small gland called the *pituitary* which is located at the base of the brain, as is the *hypothalamus* which controls the pituitary.

The hypothalamus is a regulator, producing hormone-releasing agents (chemicals), and these stimulate the pituitary to produce its own hormones. Acting as a control centre, the hypothalamus has a complex 'feedback' relationship between a woman's mind and her body, and can be affected by both her emotions and her physical state. It will respond by reducing the production of releasing agents if either, or both, is under stress.

Stress

Stress can play a considerable part when a woman's periods become heavier, irregular or painful. For instance, her periods can cease altogether or, paradoxically, become heavier through a change of circumstances, such as the death of a loved one, marital breakdown, moving house or travelling. Pain can also be evident, but it is more than just a 'pain' – it is also an interwoven number of symptoms ranging from cramps, lower abdominal pain and backache to stomach upsets and violent headaches. Not for nothing do many women regard their periods as a 'curse', especially if they are constantly away from work, suffer intolerable pain with sexual intercourse, as well as the embarrassment in public of finding blood on the back of clothing.

Diagnosis and treatment

The doctor will need to ascertain the length and intervals of periods and duration of excessive bleeding, as well as taking any bleeding between periods and bleeding after sexual intercourse into account.

Any method of contraception will be checked as some intra-uterine devices are associated with excessive menstrual bleeding. There will be a pelvic examination by the doctor and a full blood count taken to check for anaemia – this is a deficiency in the haemoglobin (oxygen) in the blood or in the number of red blood cells. Symptoms of anaemia include tiredness, extreme or unnatural paleness and lack of energy. Anaemia is likely to result from continual very heavy periods and, for some women, it can be alleviated by iron tablets.

Providing there is no evidence of pelvic abnormality, the woman will be offered drug therapy: this can either be non-hormonal, such as mefenamic acid which can reduce blood loss by an average of 50 per cent, or hormonal drugs such as danazol.

Drug therapy may provide only temporary or intermittent relief, or there might be unacceptable side-effects, so surgery could be indicated and the woman therefore referred to a consultant.

Surgery

A common minor surgical procedure called a D & C (dilation and curettage) may well be suggested: the purpose of this is to take samples of the endometrium (lining of the uterus) for examination under a microscope, as they may reveal the causes of excessive menstrual bleeding, bleeding between periods, bleeding during and after sex, and after the menopause.

Unfortunately, for many years a D & C has been considered a therapeutic procedure for curing menstrual disorders, but it is only a diagnostic tool and, while the first period after a D & C is lighter than previously, subsequent periods are not. When this happens, the consultant is likely to recommend a hysterectomy as the only solution to menorrhagia.

> *By the time I was referred to a consultant I was having very heavy periods which lasted for ten days in a cycle of 21 days.* Cathryn (Dorset)

> *I needed blood transfusions at least every six weeks for four years because of persistent uncontrolled bleeding.* Marea (Fife)

> *The bleeding was so profuse that on some days I had to wear babies' disposable nappies to just walk a short way to pick up my children from school.* Lyn (London)

Fibroids

These are lumps of fibrous and muscular tissue found growing on all levels of the uterus, although they have also been discovered in other areas within the pelvis.

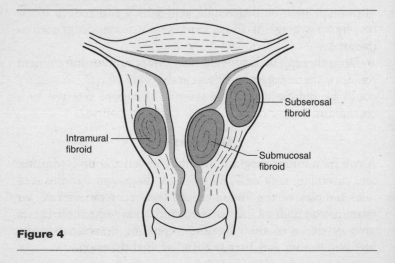

Figure 4

Most women over the age of 30 have got at least one fibroid and they occur either singly or in large numbers. They rarely become malignant (i.e. turn cancerous) but tend to get bigger and may reach the size of a seven-month pregnancy. They are known to shrink naturally in women near their menopause. Some fibroids cause problems, others do not, and the reasons for this are unknown at present, although some researchers believe that fibroids are sensitive to oestrogen and are more likely to grow when high levels of this hormone are present.

Small fibroids often cause no problems and indeed many women are unaware that they have any unless they have a gynaecological examination. No treatment will be necessary, although the doctor will want to check their size regularly.

Symptoms

Small fibroids can continue to grow, sometimes very slowly, and many women become accustomed to a gradual onset of problems which are tolerated until there is persistent discomfort. They therefore need to be aware that any of the following symptoms in their menstrual cycles could indicate that fibroids are growing and require further investigation:

- Heavy and painful periods
- Painful periods with large blood clots
- Abdominal, pelvic and/or back pain
- Pressure on the bladder and frequent urination
- An increase in stomach and waist size
- Profound fatigue
- Painful and uncomfortable sexual intercourse

Diagnosis

After examination by a consultant, an ultrasound scan may be carried out. This is a painless diagnostic technique in which the pelvic organs are viewed on a video monitor. A clear picture of the uterus is created and this will show the size and position of the fibroids, although ultrasound cannot determine how deeply they have invaded the uterus.

Treatment

In younger women who hope to have children, the fibroids can be removed by a surgical procedure called *myomectomy* which is carried out under general anaesthesia in hospital. This is a difficult operation because it involves shelling out the fibroid swellings and closing the surfaces with large stitches of soluble catgut. Fibroids within the uterus can be removed by resectoscope (a surgical instrument used for endometrial resection when the lining of the uterus is cut away).

If the woman does not wish to retain her fertility but does want to keep her uterus, small fibroids can be treated by endometrial resection or endometrial ablation (removal of the endometrium using either heat generated by a powerful laser beam or energy similar to that used in microwave ovens).

Hysterectomy is recommended when fibroids are very large and troublesome and research shows that 37 per cent of hysterectomies performed in the United Kingdom are for this complaint.

> *A period for me meant three days of cramps in my lower abdomen and thighs followed by a flow of such proportion that I resorted to disposable nappies for protection as towels. Even the maternity sanitary towels were useless . . . I am now a changed woman after the operation for fibroids.* Ann (Clwyd)

> *The reason for my operation was a fibroid which had grown to the size of a small football and caused me to have a period lasting 24 days.* Sandra (Shrewsbury)

Endometriosis

This is a disease affecting many women in their reproductive years and, as yet, nobody in the medical profession knows exactly why it occurs. It is a progressive chronic condition with acute episodes, and is the reason for 6 per cent of hysterectomies in the United Kingdom.

The cells that form the endometrium (lining of the uterus)

develop outside their normal location, so that instead of being part of the tissue of the endometrium, the cells form little clusters of tissue outside the uterus.

These bits of misplaced tissue are called endometrial implants, and they respond to the monthly stimulation of the woman's ovarian hormones during menstruation – they build up, break down and bleed as if they were still within the uterus. Sometimes patches of endometrial implants rupture during menstruation, spreading more cells to other surfaces within the pelvis so that new spots of endometriosis develop.

However, unlike the lining of the uterus which is expelled from the woman's body through the vagina during menstruation, the blood and tissue sloughed off by the endometrial implants have nowhere to go. This results in internal bleeding and degeneration of the blood and tissue, which inflames the surrounding area and leads to the formation of scar tissue. The areas of scar tissue form adhesions: these are thick bands of scar tissue that can form after surgery, and are often the result of the use of catgut and clamps and rough handling of tissue. Adhesions can extend from one organ to another so that they get stuck together.

A consequence of this is that an obstruction is created which prevents an organ functioning normally: for instance, a Fallopian tube can adhere in such a way that the open end is unable to move nearer the ovary at ovulation.

One of the most distressing aspects of the disease is that it can result in infertility as endometriosis is often diagnosed only after a woman has spent many years trying to conceive. If pregnancy can be achieved, the disease will disappear and this can continue for months or even years after the woman has had the child, but may reappear again.

Symptoms

Results of a survey of endometriosis sufferers undertaken in 1991 by the Endometriosis Society (now the National Endometriosis Society) reported the following major symptoms:

- Severely painful periods
- Painful ovulation
- Swollen abdomen
- Depression, tiredness and lethargy
- Loss of large blood clots during periods
- Painful sex
- Painful defecation
- Constipation

Another form of endometriosis is *adenomyosis*, sometimes called 'internal endometriosis' because the endometrial tissue invades the deeper muscle layers of the uterus, causing the uterus to expand every time a woman has a period. Again, the degenerating blood and tissue cannot escape and continues to accumulate inside. Although women with adenomyosis may have symptoms such as very painful periods, heavy bleeding and severe back pain, there are no symptoms that are peculiar to this disease alone, and it is often only diagnosed after a hysterectomy.

Diagnosis

Endometriosis is hard to diagnose, especially in the early stages, as many of the symptoms of endometriosis coincide with what women (and their doctors) often expect as a 'normal' part of being a woman (e.g. painful periods). It is generally recognised that women with a history of secondary or acquired dysmenorrhoea, i.e. progressive pain before, during and/or after a period, painful intercourse, pelvic pain and infertility, should be considered for investigation for endometriosis.

The only sure way to detect the disease is by a minor operation called a *laparoscopy* which is performed under anaesthetic. The surgeon makes a tiny incision through the abdomen and pumps it up with carbon dioxide gas in order to separate the organs from the abdominal wall. A small lighted tube (laparoscope) is inserted through the incision, allowing the surgeon a full view of the pelvic cavity. This shows where the implants are growing and how extensive the scar tissue and adhesions have become.

Some surgeons remove all the visible deposits of endometriotic tissue by laser at the same time as making the diagnosis, and laparoscopic instruments are used to separate adhesions. However, endometrial implants may be hidden among the tissues, or the pelvic adhesions may be too dense for the laparoscope to give a clear view of the pelvic organs, so a further surgical procedure may be required.

● If you decide to undergo hysterectomy and are worried about the possibility of adhesions, contact the Adhesions Helpline (see Useful Addresses, page 148).

Treatment

This depends on the age of the woman and her wish to remain fertile, as well as the severity of the disease and how far it has progressed.

Extensive endometriosis can be assessed by means of a major operation called a *laparotomy* (opening of the abdomen) when an incision is made just below the bikini line. The surgeon removes the endometrial implants, separates the adhesions and attempts to conserve or improve reproductive capacity. This operation might follow straight after an investigation by laparoscopy so the woman would be asked to give her formal consent to any surgery before the laparoscopy, as she would not regain consciousness between the two procedures.

However, this form of surgery is often not sufficient to control endometriosis, as new implants may occur and very small spots remain. Drug treatments which aim to stop the monthly cycles, thereby inhibiting the growth and bleeding of the endometrial implants, are prescribed by the woman's doctor, but side-effects can sometimes be a problem.

While there is ovarian function, endometriosis can recur. Surgery involving hysterectomy and removal of the ovaries is the only permanent cure if severe symptoms persist and all other treatments have been tried.

My health problems started two years before my hysterectomy. At the time I had a woman GP who told me repeatedly that my symptoms – sudden painful periods after years of pain-free ones, constant low backache, spotting between periods, low stomach ache for three weeks out of four, and large blood clots – were all due to my age. I was 38. Christine (Kelvedon)

Pelvic Inflammatory Disease (PID)

Common infections in the pelvis affect many women. Most of these are not serious and are contained at the entrance of or inside the vagina. They only cause grave problems when affecting the uterus, the Fallopian tubes or the ovaries, and irreversible damage can result if effective treatment is not given in time to stop the disease spreading. Often there is a gynaecological history of treatment for ovarian cysts and bladder infections, and PID is most commonly found in the aftermath of sexually transmitted diseases such as chlamydia.

Symptoms

There is severe abdominal pain, a high temperature and an offensive-smelling discharge from the vagina. Pain may be experienced during sexual intercourse or menstruation, the latter may become irregular and the blood loss heavier.

Treatment

A cure by drugs is possible if antibiotics are given early on and consistently until all signs of the infection have cleared. This could mean a couple of courses over months, or even two years of drug treatment.

Destroying the infection more directly by surgical removal of the diseased parts – ovaries, Fallopian tubes and uterus – may be a preferred choice, and approximately 3 per cent of hysterectomies are performed for PID.

At 18 I developed an ovarian cyst which was ruptured by a doctor because of too rough an examination. I was left with some internal bleeding before they operated and this left me with severe adhesions. Five months later I developed another cyst and this time I also had my right ovary removed. Six months afterwards I had a cyst on my left ovary, and during the following seven years I had endless pelvic infections and pain – also two healthy babies and three miscarriages. Yet another operation for an ovarian cyst was carried out. Finally I couldn't cope any longer with the pain and frequent hospital admissions, so I had my hysterectomy last March. It had been put off for two years because of my age (I am 28 years old). After about six months I now feel really well. Annette (Brunei)

Prolapse

Prolapse simply means something coming down. A prolapse of the uterus means the uterus has dropped due to a weakening of the ligaments which support it. The uterus can descend straight down one-third, two-thirds or even the entire length of the vagina, or it can descend at an angle – forwards, so that it presses on the bladder, or backwards, pressing on the bowel and rectum (back passage).

A uterine prolapse tends to happen during a woman's middle years. The muscles and ligaments often weaken at that time anyway and this is compounded by the secretion of lower levels of the female sex hormone (oestrogen) during and after the menopause. Thus there is a loss of strength and elasticity and the tissues become thin and stretched.

Symptoms

These include:

- 'Dragging' sensations and heaviness in the lower abdomen
- Feeling the need to pass urine very suddenly (urge incontinence) or passing small quantities when coughing, laughing or sneezing (stress incontinence)
- Feeling that 'something is falling out'
- Difficulty achieving penetration during sexual intercourse
- Constipation.

Treatment

This depends on the degree of prolapse. If it is mild, the doctor will suggest improvements in lifestyle, such as losing weight, regular exercise and additional fibre (roughage) in the diet. Hormone replacement therapy may also be prescribed.

Hysterectomy is recommended when there is a severe prolapse and is the reason for 6 per cent of hysterectomies in the United Kingdom. It may be combined with repair surgery to the vagina, bladder or bowel.

> *My painful and heavy periods appeared to get worse during the 18 months before the hysterectomy for a prolapse, and I felt really ill during those times. The operation revealed a mass of fibroids which had elongated the uterus, causing it to prolapse.* Margaret (Cambridge)

> *The awful dragging feeling, vaginal discomfort and backache have now gone.* Elizabeth (Andover)

Cancer

Most women feel overwhelmed when told they have cancer. Many different emotions arise which can cause confusion and frequent changes of mood.

The most immediate reaction is shock and disbelief – 'I can't believe it, it can't be true' – and it may be difficult for some to talk about the illness with family and friends, while others feel a constant urge to discuss it with those around them. Once it is believed, fear and uncertainty arise: 'Am I going to die? Will I be in pain?' In fact, nowadays many cancers are curable if caught at an early stage and a great number of cancer patients experience no pain at all.

Partners can often find it difficult to express their own fears and anxieties, yet bringing these out into the open is just as important, particularly if one outcome of the cancer is a loss of potential parenthood.

Between 5 per cent and 10 per cent of hysterectomies in the United Kingdom are for cancer of the reproductive organs and these concern the cervix, ovary and uterus.

Cancer of the Cervix

Cancer of the cervix or 'neck of the womb' is the only cancer at present which can be prevented through the detection of cell abnormalities after a smear test. Worldwide, cancer of the cervix is the second most common female cancer, and very high incidence rates have been recorded in countries such as China, Latin America and the Caribbean.

It develops from a pre-cancerous condition known as CIN, and at that stage the pre-cancer is entirely confined to the surface layers of skin on the cervix. If abnormalities are found at this stage these pre-cancerous changes are 100 per cent curable. If undetected, the fully developed cancer invades the tissue below the skin surfaces and develops a tendency to spread by the drainage channels of the cervix out towards the side of the pelvis.

There is now conclusive evidence that cervical cancer is caused by a sexually transmitted virus, yet some research also indicates that the environment and heredity play a part. Early age at the time of first sexual intercourse and multiple partners (often these two factors go together) are high risk factors, and the risk for a woman is raised with the number of sexual contacts her partner has had.

Symptoms

Bleeding is the most common symptom. This may appear as altered periods, usually heavier or irregular, or as bleeding between periods, particularly after sexual intercourse, and bleeding after the menopause. There may be an offensive-smelling discharge due to infection in the surface of the cancer.

Treatment

This will depend on how advanced the cancer is found to be, but if it is invasive (i.e. it has spread) then there is no option but a *radical hysterectomy*. This differs from an ordinary hysterectomy in that it is more extensive and complex to perform, and, as there are fewer doctors with these additional necessary skills, the woman may well have to be referred to a more appropriate centre for the operation.

In a radical hysterectomy, known as Wertheim's hysterectomy, the uterus is removed together with the cervix and the cancer. In order to be sure that the cancer is cleared, a wide band of normal tissue must also be taken away, which means the loss of the top half of the vagina too, plus the tissue stretching out to the bony part of the pelvis. The glands on the side wall of the pelvis are removed and sent for examination by a pathologist.

In younger women (under 45 years) the ovaries can be retained, so that although menstruation will cease, the female hormone (oestrogen) will continue to be produced and there will be no symptoms of an early menopause (change of life).

I am one of five sisters, and because of what had happened to my mother – she had a hysterectomy for cervical cancer when she was 29 – she made us all have regular smear tests. Thank goodness she did . . . I also developed cervical cancer and, after the operation, felt as though a great black cloud had been lifted from me. I looked at life so differently. Sue (Dorset)

Being alive and watching my daughter grow up are the bonuses for having had a hysterectomy for cervical cancer. Suzanne (Bradford)

Despite an increase in cases of cancer of the cervix, there was a reduction in the number of deaths in 1992 (1,860) from those recorded in 1988 (2,000). It should not kill one single woman. It is eminently preventable.

Cancer of the Ovary

Ovarian cancer is the most common gynaecological cancer in women in the United Kingdom. It is predominantly a disease of older, post-menopausal women, with 90 per cent of cases occurring after the age of 45 years. Worldwide, the highest rates are recorded in white Caucasian women in northern Europe and North America, and the lowest rates in Indian, Japanese and Chinese women.

The position of the ovaries deep within the abdomen acts against early diagnosis and there are still no reliable screening tests. It grows relatively silently within the pelvis and abdomen without the woman noticing any major alterations in health. Often the diagnosis is not made until the cancer has grown to a very large size or even spread widely, thus making cure difficult.

Symptoms

These are often vague. Bowel upsets, nausea, indigestion, pelvic discomfort, menstrual upsets, backache, feelings of pressure, dragging sensations and even breathlessness have been described, as has an increase in waist size without any real increase in weight, and weight loss.

Any symptoms that occur develop because the cancer presses on structures close to the abdomen. These include the bladder (feelings of wanting to pass urine or causing the woman to pass frequent small quantities of urine), and the bowel (causing a desire to empty the bowel but with little result), or alternatively constipation, or diarrhoea if the cancer irritates the bowel.

It is very important that the woman's doctor take the symptoms seriously and that she is referred for a specialist gynaecological opinion.

Diagnosis

At hospital, the woman's vagina, abdomen and neck of the uterus will be examined fully. The specialist will be feeling for cysts (swellings filled with fluid) in the abdomen and glands and in the neck of the uterus. If there is a large cyst in the abdomen, the specialist will be able to make a confident diagnosis that there is a cyst of the ovary. Unfortunately, it is impossible at this stage to be certain the tumour (or abnormal growth) is cancerous. Any doubts about the presence of a cyst would be resolved by an ultrasound scan.

Treatment

If a cyst is found, the woman will be admitted to hospital for a laparoscopy. This allows the ovaries to be viewed directly and for tissue samples to be removed and analysed straight away to find out if they are benign or malignant. If it is found to be a benign fluid-filled cyst, then this can be drained away using a fine needle and no further treatment will be needed.

Another diagnostic procedure is a laparotomy, which involves opening the abdomen to assess the problem; any necessary surgery would then be carried out. If this follows a laparoscopy, the woman would be asked to give her formal consent to any surgery before undergoing laparoscopy.

Extensive surgery may be required if a malignant tumour is found – a hysterectomy to remove the uterus, removal of the Fallopian tubes and both ovaries, as well as any particles of cancer which lie on other organs.

However, the operation can form only part of the treatment: it may be complemented by the use of chemotherapy (drug treatment) to deal with any microscopic cells which may have been left behind, and this drug treatment has to be carefully monitored. It has a tendency to make the patient feel sick and low, and the treatment takes a long time. Mentally, this cancer is very demanding. It is not unusual to feel tired, irritable and depressed, and the woman may find she has no appetite or enjoyment of food, as well as no interest in sex, until the drug treatment is completed.

As I had just received my second dose of chemotherapy, I was not over the moon to be told the prognosis was not good – I understand that ovarian cancer kills 4,000 women a year so I'm lucky that after 15 months, all appears to be going well for me. Valerie (Buckinghamshire)

I had ovarian cancer when I was 34 (I am now 40) and don't feel the operation was that bad compared with the emotional scars – my inability to bear children has caused me years of anguish. Janet (London)

Cancer of the Body of the Uterus

This cancer generally occurs after the woman's periods have stopped naturally (after the menopause) although it can also occur in younger women. It is usually a cancer of the glandular tissue in the lining of the body of the uterus. Sometimes there are rarer cancers in the muscular part of the uterus.

Symptoms

As this cancer tends to develop after the menopause, the most important symptom is the renewal of bleeding. All vaginal bleeding after periods have apparently ceased should be thoroughly investigated.

There are very few other symptoms, so it is doubly important not to ignore this bleeding. Pelvic discomfort, backache, feelings of pressure and dragging sensations may be experienced, but these symptoms are not specific for this disease.

For the woman who is still menstruating, a major alteration in menstrual pattern should also be taken seriously and fully investigated.

Treatment

Outpatient pelvic examination by a specialist cannot reveal what is happening within the cavity of the uterus, so a D & C will be carried out in hospital. Samples of the endometrium (lining of the uterus) will be taken and sent for analysis by a pathologist.

If this analysis reveals a cancer, the woman will be recalled as it will be necessary to have further treatment, probably a hysterectomy.

The first surgeon in the UK to perform a hysterectomy for cancer was James Blundell, Physician at Guy's Hospital, London. It was performed on 19 February 1828 and the patient was 50-year old Mary Moulden who had suffered for seven months from daily uterine haemorrhage.

Finally, a hysterectomy can be the only solution for a haemorrhage which proves impossible to stop. Sometimes, during childbirth, events occur which lead to abnormally large bleeds, and a hysterectomy can be the only way to save a woman's life. But the shock to both the woman and her partner can be traumatic, as 30-year-old Barbara (from Reading) described when she found herself with a baby born by Caesarean section and post-partum haemorrhage.

There was no time to adjust to what would happen and very little time to talk about my feelings with the midwives. I also had to hide my feelings from my husband as he was unable to cope with my emotions, mainly because I was in hospital for six weeks and he was under extra pressure as the nanny never got up at night to see to our daughter of 19 months – he was frightened of saying too much for fear of the nanny leaving.

Taking Time to Consider

If hysterectomy is recommended for non-malignant reasons, that is, other than for cancer – the woman should ask herself the following questions:

1. Are my symptoms so unbearable as to make my life a continuing misery?
2. Do I still hope to bear children?
3. Am I sure hysterectomy is the right solution for me?
4. Do I understand what is involved?
   and
5. Are there any alternative treatments available?

It is these alternative treatments which we shall consider in the next chapter.

Chapter Two
Part 1
A Change of Emphasis

Women today are undergoing more menstrual cycles. Not only is the age of a girl's first period dropping (from an average of 18 a century ago to 13 today) but there is also far less child-bearing and breast-feeding, both of which inhibit menstruation.

During her reproductive life, today's woman will experience 400 or more periods. This is a far cry from an average of 35 periods experienced by her grandmother or great-grandmother when one pregnancy followed another, almost at annual intervals, and families of ten or more children were commonplace.

Very few of today's women will escape menstrual disorders. Over 10 per cent of all visits by women to their general practitioner are for menstrual problems, and that represents, in primary health care alone, a cost to the UK in excess of £250 million per annum. The costs in terms of well-being as an adolescent/employee/partner/parent are as impossible to calculate as are the loss of earnings and additional personal expenditure.

Menstrual loss

The amount of blood women lose each month varies enormously from individual to individual and, in addition, stressful occurrences can change the pattern of the monthly cycle. Because of this wide variation between women, it is impossible to define or describe a 'normal' period and, as a consequence, there are very few guidelines to help define what is 'normal' and what is 'abnormal' in terms of the amount, length and frequency of bleeding. However, for any individual woman the amount of blood lost every month tends to remain relatively constant, apart from slight variations with age. As a result of this relative constancy, each woman tends to see her own periods as 'normal for her', regardless of how much blood she loses each month.

So if you feel your periods have become heavier, you are defining them in comparison with your 'normal' blood loss. But again, because this varies enormously from woman to woman, it may be the case that your heavier bleeding is still actually lighter than that which other women would consider to be 'normal'.

Heavy periods are defined by doctors as the loss of more than 80 ml of blood during any one period, and it is considered excessive when:

- a pad or tampon has to be changed more often than every two hours, and
- more than ten pads or tampons are used each day for more than seven days.

If you are already sure you cannot cope with your unexplained and increased blood loss, there are two possible courses of action – you may be referred immediately to a gynaecologist, or your doctor may prescribe a course of non-hormonal treatment (such as mefenamic acid) or hormonal treatment (such as Danazol). The main problem with these is that they affect different women in different ways. Some find that their bleeding is gradually reduced, others feel no change and a few women's problems become worse. If this treatment is ineffective, surgery is indicated.

For years, this has meant hysterectomy. That alternatives to this operation have come about during the last two decades is a demonstration of the advances in medical technology coupled with the imagination and courage of pioneering medical specialists.

In the Beginning . . .

In 1981, 11 women with intractable uterine bleeding resistant to medical treatment were admitted to Yale New Haven Hospital, Connecticut, USA. Emergency hysterectomies appeared to be the only way of saving their lives. But the chances of surviving a major operation were unlikely for most of them as the group consisted of three patients with leukaemia, six patients who were extreme anaesthesia risks (four alcoholics and two drug addicts) and two who refused definitive surgical therapy.

One of the gynaecologists, Alan DeCherney, came up with an idea: if a man's prostate gland could be removed by 'burning it', perhaps the same technique could be used on a woman's endometrium (the lining of the uterus which gives rise to menstrual bleeding). He tried, using the identical instrument, a resectoscope. The bleeding stopped.

What the surgeon had done was to confirm a way of permanently disrupting the basic mechanism of a woman's periods by the surgical removal of the endometrium.

Here at last was a real alternative to hysterectomy, or so it was thought, especially as medical technology grasped the opportunity to develop its potential, and provided the surgical marketplace with further necessary hardware for this minimally invasive surgical treatment.

There was an enthusiastic response from many gynaecologists in the United Kingdom in the mid-1980s. However, surgeons experienced a sharp learning curve as more realistic expectations for its success rate replaced the exaggerated hopes of its pioneers – many found the treatment was difficult to perform and gave unexpected complications. These were investigated in the MISTLETOE survey (Minimally Invasive Surgical Techniques: Laser, EndoThermal Or Endoresection survey) which examined the complications of TCRE, laser, rollerball, radiofrequency and cryoablation as applied to 10,686 women. **Published in 1997, it concluded that the safest treatments were TCRE using rollerball, or laser.**

Confidence increased as experienced practitioners obtained successful results, and this is evinced in research studies from

1995 onwards. Some of these involved relatively few women, such as the one in 1999 concerning 204 women who joined a randomised comparison of endometrial ablation with hysterectomy four to five years previously. **It found that 76 per cent of women with dysfunctional uterine bleeding who underwent endometrial ablation avoided a hysterectomy.**

The discovery in 1981 that some abnormal menstruation could be managed in a less traumatic way has brought relief to thousands of women. The following are treatments which offer a viable alternative to hysterectomy.

Transcervical Resection of the Endometrium (TCRE)

The first step is the inspection of the uterine cavity via the vagina and cervix by means of a thin telescope (hysteroscope). This is a viewing instrument no thicker than a pencil and it allows the surgeon a good view inside because it has a light and a telescopic lens.

The surgeon needs to be sure that the uterus is essentially normal. If there are any fibroids (benign growths in the wall of the uterus), they must be small. Different surgery would be needed if they were large or if there were evidence of endometriosis. Once the surgeon is satisfied that it is in order to carry out the surgical procedure, a resectoscope is used. This is similar to a hysteroscope but in addition to the telescope there is a small wire loop at the end. When an electric current is passed through this wire loop, segments of the endometrium are reamed away until the underlying muscle is seen. Many surgeons then replace the wire loop with a roller-ball electrode to destroy certain areas of the uterus which are more susceptible to uterine perforation. Some of the tissue is sent for analysis to ensure that no disease is present.

Periods will stop completely if you choose to have a total resection. A partial resection can be carried out which results in light periods.

Period pain

TCRE can reduce or eradicate menstrual bleeding but will not necessarily abolish period pain. When it does not, the intensity and duration of the pain appears to be tolerable, partly because it can be controlled by painkilling tablets and partly because of the overall improvement in the quality of life. If the pain worsens after TCRE the doctor should be consulted, as an investigation might become necessary.

Outcome of TCRE

Most of the women who wrote to me about their experience of TCRE were delighted with the results.

I opened my own florist shop the week after the operation (in fact, I had the operation on the Friday and was painting the shop on Saturday). I now work six days a week with a 3.30 a.m. start for three mornings, and I certainly couldn't have contemplated this at all with the previous problems I had with my periods. Maxine (Oxford).

If I start my period on a Monday morning, it is finished by Tuesday afternoon. After years of my periods lasting ten days I now think I'm very lucky, and it is always pain-free. It has totally changed my life. Margaret (Royston).

I am not filled with dread at the thought of more soiled sheets, disturbed nights and having to wear black or navy skirts for a few days. Glenna (London).

Now I no longer take iron tablets or spend a fortune at the chemist's. Gillian (Bedford).

I don't know how long I will feel so much better (I had fibroids and they may grow back). Julie (Paisley).

This is a superb alternative to hysterectomy, which would have been like using a sledgehammer to crack a nut. Jane (Oxford).

However, there were a few women for whom the operation was only partially successful:

After two years I had a sudden bleed, which was quite a shock, and I went on to have a hysterectomy. Sylvia (London).

My periods stopped for six months and then restarted. Marilyn (London).

I have a slight bleed for one to two days and the only problem is the severe pain. Toyin (London).

I have gained weight since surgery and experienced even more severe PMT. Frances (Taunton).

Hysteroscopic Endometrial Ablation with a Laser (Heal)

This operative procedure is similar to that of TCRE except that a powerful laser beam is used to vaporise the endometrium.

The laser is introduced into the uterus through the hysteroscope and, under direct vision, as much of the endometrium as possible is destroyed – literally 'at the speed of light'. The idea is to cut down the bleeding as much as possible, but some slight menstrual bleeding may be experienced after treatment as it is not always possible to destroy every part of the endometrium.

The patient is asked to take a drug (possibly Danazol) for four to six weeks beforehand: this shrinks the endometrium so that the laser is more effective. Periods may cease while this drug is being taken.

Periods do not necessarily stop completely after laser treatment but some women are able to accept this because the intensity of symptoms, such as feeling bloated or pain, are greatly reduced.

The first laser treatment stopped the very heavy bleeding but my periods lasted around a week and occurred every three weeks. I was offered a repeat treatment as there was some evidence of live tissue on the part of my uterus which was the last area to receive the laser. The second laser treatment was completed successfully and I have had no further bleeding. Cathy (Edinburgh).

In the year since my laser therapy, I have lost a stone in weight, given up painkillers and set up in business for myself. I have no periods, some mild PMT and my own GP describes me as a 'new woman' and can't believe the change in me. Christine (Ayr).

From Surgery to Recovery

The patient could be in hospital for between one and three days. Patients who have to travel a long way would probably be asked to come in for the night before treatment. In some cases, patients are in before breakfast and out for supper.

No food or drink is taken for about four hours before surgery, as a full anaesthetic is likely to be given. Preparation for this surgery is minimal: the patient changes into a surgical gown, a sedative or injection is given to aid relaxation and induce sleepiness, and the patient is then taken to the operating theatre where a general anaesthetic is administered.

The patient's legs are supported apart by stirrups and the vaginal area thoroughly cleaned with antiseptic. An extensive local anaesthetic is injected into the cervix, which is then widened using metal or plastic rods, and the hysteroscope is inserted. If the treatment is TCRE, a fluid is run into the womb and out again via the hysteroscope – this keeps the view clear during surgery.

The whole procedure takes between 15 and 30 minutes, after which the patient spends time in the recovery room. Once the anaesthetic has worn off, the patient can either go home or return to the hospital ward. Painkilling tablets are offered, to be taken as and when necessary. Most patients feel a little shaky and, if discharged from hospital on the same day, should not drive immediately afterwards.

Pain and discomfort

The uterus is a muscular structure and responds to pain and heat with a cramping sensation. This can be extremely intense and may temporarily be very painful. It can be focused above the pubic bone or in the lower back. The experience and degree of pain vary from woman to woman, so they are difficult to predict.

Recovering at home

Patterns of discomfort over the first few days vary: sometimes an increase in uterine pain can be an indication of over-exertion, so a decrease in activity is necessary. Although actual hospitalisation has been brief, an operative procedure has been carried out so it is important to rest and allow time for the body to heal. Extreme fatigue is frequently the most difficult symptom that occurs; although some women resume normal activities immediately afterwards, others need longer to recover.

Advantages of these Treatments

- They involve minor surgery with no abdominal incision and resulting scars.
- The time spent in hospital ranges from one to three days.
- Convalescence is usually between one and two weeks.
- The uterus is retained.
- They may be suitable for women who have increased risk factors for major surgery, for example women with severe heart disease, extreme anaesthesia risks, major respiratory difficulties and blood disorders.

Disadvantages of these Treatments

- Complications from fluid overload, infections, uterine perforations and injury to surrounding organs can cause morbidity and even mortality.

- The outcome of some complications could be further surgery, i.e. bowel repair and hysterectomy.
- They are not suitable for all cases of heavy bleeding, i.e. where large fibroids or endometriosis are present.
- Menstrual bleeding can be eradicated or reduced but period pain will not necessarily be abolished.
- They are not recommended for women who want children. Pregnancies have occurred following treatment and it is believed there is a higher risk of miscarriage.

Uterine Thermal Balloon Therapy (ThermaChoice)

Although not part of the MISTLETOE study, other surgical alternatives to hysterectomy for menorrhagia have evolved during the last 20 years. Foremost amongst these is uterine thermal balloon therapy.

This simplified method of endometrial ablation was developed in 1994 in order to solve some of the problems experienced by even skilled surgeons when undertaking TCRE and laser. No specialised training is required of the gynaecologist as the procedure is similar to that of inserting an intra-uterine contraceptive device (IUD). It is now available in 58 hospitals in the United Kingdom.

Operative procedure

A fine catheter with a deflated latex balloon at one end is inserted into the uterus. The balloon is inflated and filled with around 10 ml of sterile fluid which expands to fit the shape and size of the uterus. This fluid is heated to 87°C for eight minutes while the endometrium is treated. Once the treatment cycle is complete and the fluid is drained away the balloon is deflated, withdrawn and discarded with the catheter.

The endometrium will be shed like a period over the next seven to ten days. Worldwide, over 45,000 women have benefited from this treatment without any serious complications. Clinical data indicate a decrease to normal bleeding or less at 12 months after treatment by 84 per cent of patients.

Advantages of this Treatment

- No instrument comes into contact with the endometrium, simply heat, and there is thus minimal blood loss.
- Local anaesthesia is usually adequate. This should be particularly advantageous for women who suffer adverse reactions to general anaesthesia, as well as those with severe medical disease.
- There is no need for hospitalisation, simply rest under supervised care in out-patient recovery for two to four hours following the procedure.

Disadvantages of this Treatment

- Clinical data show that up to 15 per cent of patients may not respond to this therapy and could require additional treatment.
- Its use appears restricted to women with a normal uterine cavity and therefore excludes women with fibroids.
- The procedure may pose some rare, but possible, safety risks. These include blood loss, perforation or rupture of the wall of the uterus, or leakage of heated fluid from the balloon into the cervix or vagina.
- Blood or tissue may collect in the uterus and/or Fallopian tubes during the months post-procedure, and may require an outpatients' procedure to correct the problem.

Two years ago my periods were appalling, and I was desperate, but didn't want a hysterectomy. So when the gynaecologist asked if I'd like to take part in clinical trials at the hospital, I jumped at the chance. I was quite sore afterwards, as though I was burning inside, but that soon passed. I no longer have periods – what a relief! Sue (Dagenham)

It was a bit like having a D & C. There were spots of blood for three weeks afterwards, then my periods stopped completely. Maureen (Cardiff)

It's a year since I went for treatment and, although I still have periods, they don't go on as long. I can cope with them now. Tracy (Romford)

Although everything is now fine, I was in a lot of pain for about a month afterwards with burning sensations in my vagina. This meant frequent trips to the gynaecologist who was very apologetic, and prescribed creams to help. The best thing I found was sitting in a lukewarm bath, that seemed to ease it. Mary (Ilford)

After surgery I was waiting to feel unwell but it didn't happen! Oonagh (Belfast)

Microwave Endometrial Ablation

In 1994 clinical trials began at the Royal United Hospital, Bath, of a therapy named microwave endometrial ablation, which researchers and gynaecologists hoped would be a rapid, simple and safe procedure delivering precise heating to burn the endometrium using microwaves.

The energy is delivered by means of an applicator inserted into the uterus. Once in position, power is applied and the applicator is slowly withdrawn with a sweeping movement to ensure all of the endometrium is treated. It takes about two to four minutes to complete and can be carried out under general or local anaesthetic.

It was the latter which concerned some of my correspondents:

The treatment was fine but I was very ill with the anaesthetic (gas and air). I was allergic to it, so I brought all the tablets up and was then given morphine later on and had to stay in hospital overnight. Carol (Shepton Mallet)

Women should make sure they feel OK with local anaesthetic. I was dizzy and sick afterwards and was kept in overnight. Karen (Bristol)

Results of research to date are encouraging as the following confirm:

> *My periods are now very light, and only for two to three days. Great!* Susan (Devizes)

> *Having suffered ten years of heavy periods when I was constantly tired and worn out, this has changed my life. I am able to do anything, go anywhere, and have slight bleeding.* Karen (Bristol)

> *I would recommend the treatment because, after 35 years of pain and misery, I am free from the monthly torment.* Carol (Shepton Mallet)

The pain of this procedure was described by a mother of two children as:

> *No worse than a severe contraction in labour and it lasted about a minute.* Jackie (Warminster)

A watery discharge usually occurs for approximately three weeks, during a recovery time varying from one day to eight weeks.

The speed and simplicity of the procedure make it ideal for either an outpatients' procedure or a day surgery setting. The failure rate appears to be associated with the thickness of the endometrium at the time of the operation and retreatment may be necessary. **Research indicates a success rate of 83 per cent for a single treatment and a total success rate of 96 per cent including retreatment.**

Embolisation of Uterine Fibroids

For decades, the only surgical solutions to troublesome fibroids have been myomectomy (if the fibroids were small) or hysterectomy if their continuing growth caused symptoms as outlined in Chapter 1. But, as with the endometrial ablation therapy described earlier, the solution of one medical problem with a particular procedure has resulted in its application to another, for embolisation had already been used for over 20 years to treat heavy bleeding after childbirth.

In 1995, Professor J H Ravina and his colleagues in France treated 16 women aged 34–48 years whose fibroids had failed to respond to medical treatment. The size and site of the fibroids were assessed by ultrascan during the weeks preceding embolisation, and monitored at three, six and 12 months or more after embolisation. At a mean follow-up of 20 months, 11 of the 16 patients reported that their symptoms had resolved, three had partial improvement and two failures required surgery (one a myomectomy, the other a hysterectomy). Ultrasound was used to assess the effect of embolisation on the fibroids and revealed a reduction of between 20–80 per cent in volume three months later. One of their patients subsequently became pregnant.

As with the ablation procedures in the early 1980s, this one has been enthusiastically adopted by medical specialists on the basis that it appears to work and is less invasive than surgery. But the current body of research is quite limited, and long-term follow-up data is not yet available.

What is encouraging in the research is the high degree of therapeutic success indicating a rate in excess of 80 per cent. Coupled with few complications, the procedure offers a major turning-point in the treatment of a condition for which 37 per cent of hysterectomies are performed in the United Kingdom.

The procedure is now being carried out in the USA, Paris and London (the London Clinic and Guy's and St Thomas) as well as hospitals in Guildford, Hull, Glasgow, Southampton, Manchester and Cardiff.

Case Study

Lindsay, now 39 years old. Single. Occupation: Special needs teacher

'Small fibroids were discovered during a routine examination/ smear test four years ago. My periods became heavier and more prolonged, so I was prescribed Ponstan by my doctor. I was all right for a few months, but a repeat prescription was refused and I was referred to a gynaecologist. He recommended a hysterectomy, which horrified me – I hoped some day I might have children, so I wouldn't consider it.

'But my periods worsened during the next 18 months. They lasted 14–21 days, and I became weak and weary, exhausted by long and heavy periods. Also I was spending a fortune on Tampax and pads.

'Eventually, blood tests revealed I was extremely anaemic, and I lived on iron tablets and iron-rich food for six weeks until my blood count was almost normal. I again saw the gynaecologist, and the fibroids were found to have grown in size equivalent to a 24-week pregnancy. Because of this, I agreed to be placed on the 'urgent' list for a hysterectomy and was told I would be called within three to four months.

'Then a friend mentioned embolisation, and gave me the name of a consultant radiologist to contact. I discussed the treatment with him, and having established I was entitled to be referred for treatment on the NHS, I asked my doctor to do so. He and the gynaecologist expressed outright scepticism and doubt but this made me all the more determined to persist, even though by then I was rattling with pills. Without them I bled continuously, and one night I truly believed I was bleeding to death.

'At last an appointment for embolisation arrived – 18 May. The following day I received an appointment for a hysterectomy – 16 May. This was 20 months after I had been put on the 'urgent' waiting list!

'I rang the hospital and cancelled the latter appointment, then confirmed the one for embolisation.'

Embolisation Procedure

Embolisation is the obstruction of a blood vessel feeding the fibroid and, starved of its blood supply, the fibroid is therefore effectively destroyed (if small) and considerably reduced in size (if large).

Following preparation for the operation, a local anaesthetic is injected into the groin. The radiologist cuts a small nick in the skin to access the femoral artery and inserts a catheter into the artery. This is then guided (using x-ray control) into the

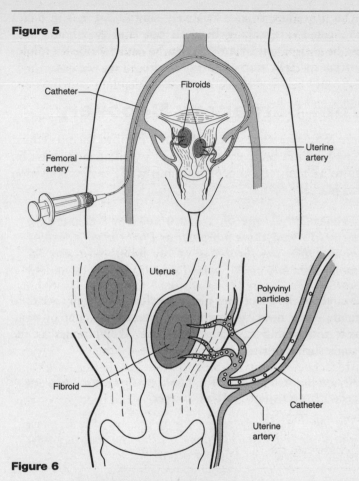

Figure 5

Catheter

Fibroids

Femoral artery

Uterine artery

Uterus

Polyvinyl particles

Fibroid

Catheter

Uterine artery

Figure 6

© The Society of Cardiovascular & Interventional Radiology www.scvir.org/fibroid

uterine artery (*Figure 5*). Once this is located, tiny grains of PVA (polyvinyl alcohol) the size of grains of sand are slowly injected via the catheter. The particles flow to the fibroids first, lodge in the blood vessels and therefore cannot travel to other parts of the body. Over several minutes, the arteries are slowly blocked, and this continues until there is an almost complete blockage of the blood flow in the multiple vessels (*Figure 6*). On completion, the other uterine artery is also embolised.

The procedure sounds relatively simple but it is in fact a complicated one, taking between one and two hours, and must be carried out by an experienced interventional radiologist (one specially trained to work with blood vessels).

From Surgery to Recovery

There is an overnight stay in hospital. Prior to the procedure, the patient will be given a sedative, as well as instruction on how to administer a morphine pump while the embolisation takes place.

> *I remember dozing off . . . waking up, and pumping away like mad at the morphine as I felt the wire pushing inside, then the throbbing of my womb – it was far worse than any period pains I'd had.* Lindsay (Swindon)

The effect of the procedure varies considerably from patient to patient: some need very strong analgesics to control pain, which will usually continue for some 12–24 hours as the fibroids shrink in size, others do not.

> *It came in waves, at times it was quite severe, but pain relief was adequate.* Moira (Exeter)

> *The pain was very severe for two days. I was given morphine but stopped taking it after the first day as it made me very sick.* Jennifer (Kent)

> *I was moderately uncomfortable afterwards but it soon passed.* Alphema (London)

> *I took oral painkillers for three to four days afterwards.* Lindsay (Swindon)

Most of my correspondents were happy with the outcome:

> *I'm really pleased I stuck to my guns and didn't have a hysterectomy, it was really worth all the hassle. The fibroid is still there, but it's so much smaller now, and*

my periods are normal. Problems such as a sensation of bloating and occasional pain ceased after six months. Lindsay (Swindon)

What a change from the past seven years, when even a half-hour bus journey was too long. Often I arrived soaked in blood to the knees. I was constantly worried about a deluge without warning, and I had to sit on plastic bags when I attended business meetings. All that is now a thing of the past and in the last six months I have become a new person (or back to the person I had almost forgotten about). My periods are short, light, almost regular. Jennifer (Kent)

It has changed my life totally and I am now full of energy. My only regret is that it took so long for the hospital to do the procedure, and during this time my fibroids greatly increased in size. Alison (Oxford)

For some there were other problems:

I do get pain in my lower abdomen from time to time, especially when my period is about to start. The most important part is I do not suffer from heavy periods any more. Mercy (London)

I still have severe pains but I can now go out when I have a period; I don't have to worry about washing lots of bloody bedclothes and I spend less money on pads. Barbara (London)

I suffered very painful, swollen legs for a time afterwards and found it difficult to climb the stairs. Marlene (Romford)

Time taken to recover varies from five days to four weeks and patients need to be aware of the following:

- Avoid standing for too long. Take things easy and rest when tired. Stay at home until really ready to go back to work.
- Avoid lifting anything heavy for the week of recovery.

- Use sanitary towels when required during the following four weeks (**not** tampons). Some vaginal bleeding may occur with the loss of small fragments of tissue, and it is common for this to include the expulsion of smaller fibroids.
- Avoid sexual intercourse for four weeks after the procedure to allow the uterus to settle down.
- If the fibroid/s are large there may be a slight elevation of temperature. Should it rise above 38°C/100.5°F, telephone the hospital where you were a patient.

Follow-up appointments at regular intervals during the following year monitor the shrinkage of fibroids.

Advantages and Disadvantages

The **advantages** of this treatment are similar to those of endometrial ablation, except that the time in hospital is usually only overnight.

The **disadvantages** centre around the following:

- Large fibroids will shrink by up to a third in size, but will not vanish. This appears well tolerated because of the return to normal menstruation. Smaller fibroids shrink completely.
- Exposure to radiation during the procedure, particularly to the ovaries. The procedure should therefore be performed only by trained interventional radiologists.
- There is a failure rate. This may be due to infection or other conditions within the pelvic region which mitigate against a successful embolisation.
- Injury to the pelvic organs is possible but none has yet been reported.

Summary

The success rates of endometrial ablation are impressive. But if you decide to undergo this treatment you need to recognise that:

- The procedure may be partially successful: some of my correspondents found their periods stopped for many years, then re-started. When this happened, some were re-treated by the same method, others tried a different type of ablation, while a minority elected to have a hysterectomy.

- The procedure may fail, for reasons that are still not fully understood.
- Having children after endometrial ablation is usually not an option.

*The impact of endometrial ablation has been considerable and it is now firmly established as a real alternative to hysterectomy for menorrhagia. **Provisional figures for 1998–1999 indicate a one-third increase in these procedures since 1993**. Uterine embolisation of fibroids demonstrates an effective method of treatment for women with this condition, albeit that it is a comparatively new procedure.*

Nearly 80 per cent of hysterectomies in the United Kingsdom are performed for menorrhagia and/or fibroids, and these two therapies offer real alternatives to major surgery.

Counselling

It is very difficult to assess accurately the amount of blood loss when a woman consults her doctor for menorrhagia, and although not available routinely, objective measurement of her menstrual blood loss (MBL) can be considered to be a vital assessment. Obtaining this measurement medically is not difficult – it involves soaking samples of a woman's sanitary devices in 5 per cent sodium hydroxide to convert the blood to alkaline haematein, the optical density of which can be measured.

In the late 1980s, 17 women aged 30–45 were recruited from the John Radcliffe Hospital gynaecology clinics, Oxford, as part of a study of menorrhagia. All had been referred for assessment with a view to hysterectomy.

Pelvic examination gave normal results and none was using hormonal or intra-uterine contraception, nor taking treatment for menstrual disorders at the time of assessment. Menstrual blood loss (MBL) was measured for two consecutive periods and the women were advised that their MBL was within normal limits (80 ml), did not constitute harm to their health and required no treatment. They were counselled individually: this covered what their blood loss was, what was normal in the population, and the risks of surgery. The women were asked why they felt their blood loss was abnormal. In addition they were offered the opportunity to contact the consultant gynaecologist, Margaret Rees, for further information and discussion if they so wished.

At a three-year follow-up, 14 of the 17 women reported that they had accepted the information and advice given and had not required any treatment for menorrhagia. Of the remaining three, two were taking mefenamic acid (which reduces MBL) and one had had a hysterectomy.

On the face of it, the results are astonishing. They indicate that thousands of hysterectomies for menorrhagia (severe menstrual bleeding) could be avoided by assessment and counselling, provided women were prepared to accept this method of treatment.

Yet a certain unease remains. Having been assessed and counselled, some of the women in this Oxford study might have felt inhibited about consulting their doctors again for menstrual problems such as period pain, cramping, backache and PMT. It might well take persistence to obtain a hysterectomy when the specialist maintained it was unnecessary. Nevertheless, the methods used in this Oxford study – assessment of MBL as well as counselling by a practice nurse – could be used by GPs before referral to a consultant. Women who perceive their blood loss to be excessive require some help, even if it does not reach the 80 ml level which clinically constitutes menorrhagia. One benefit of this approach might be to lessen the depression which has been observed in a high proportion of women on the waiting list for hysterectomy.

Chapter Two
Part 2
Fringe Benefits

Every day, hundreds of people seek the help of acupuncturists, chiropractors, osteopaths, herbalists and homoeopaths as well as practitioners of lesser-known therapies.

Why should this be so? Why is there such interest in complementary medicine, given the extraordinary achievements of orthodox medicine? It would be hard to exaggerate the benefits obtained by applying scientific principles to medicine: bacterial infections are curable, smallpox has been wiped out worldwide and polio has ceased to be a major problem, at least in Western countries. Almost every week our televisions, press and radio bring us enthusiastic accounts of new medical techniques or discoveries – organ transplantation, 'test-tube' babies, hip and knee replacements, cures for many cancers and gene therapy.

And yet . . . The fact is that much of this is divorced from the daily lives of people. For women, it is frequently menstrual disorders which badly affect their way of life, often presenting as depression, headaches, backache, water retention and PMT. The end result of an (average) six-minute interview with a harassed GP is most likely to be a prescription for anti-depressants/painkillers/tranquillisers/sleeping tablets. Some of these are helpful in the short term but many are not. They do not provide solutions and carry the potential risks of addiction and side-effects. Doctors have never tried harder and been less well loved.

Public alarm has been fuelled by the experience of the thalidomide tragedy in the late 1950s, the Opren scandal in the 1980s and addiction to prescribed drugs such as Valium. Many people are disenchanted with the lack of time given by doctors and are suspicious of drugs. This has provided fertile ground for complementary medicine.

For years, the British Medical Association (the doctors' trade union) was less than welcoming of complementary medicine – and with some justification. Anyone could rent a room, buy a leather couch, screw a shiny brass plate outside their door, preferably with a string of impressive-sounding letters after their name, and bingo! they were in business. They could be a positive menace and danger to the potential patient – but how was the patient to know that?

A poll conducted by the BBC in 1999 found that the number of people using complementary and alternative medicine had doubled over the past six years to 21 per cent of the population. Many claimed to have had their conditions cured or improved. Some of them consulted practitioners in the following three therapies – acupuncture, medical herbalism and homoeopathy – as did the many women who wrote to me about their experiences of complementary therapy.

Acupuncture

The use of acupuncture caught the Western imagination around 1958 when it became renowned for its effectiveness in pain control, primarily for post-operative care. Later, it was introduced as anaesthesia during operations, starting with minor ones such as tooth extraction and progressing to major operations on the limbs and abdomen.

Unfortunately, this dramatic use of acupuncture led to a widespread misconception about the effectiveness of what is probably the oldest surviving medical discipline, going back to periods before recorded history, and there is very little doubt it was in China that acupuncture was first used widely.

The whole theory of Chinese medicine evolved out of an era of philosophical speculation and intense consideration of the nature of life by great thinkers such as Confucius. Its four methods of diagnosis – Observing; Listening and Smelling;

Asking; and Touching – remain as much the cornerstones of modern-day acupuncture treatment as they did circa 200BC when a Chinese doctor, Bia Que, brought a prince out of a coma by acupuncture. (Legend has it that acupuncture was first discovered by a soldier shot by an arrow who found, when struck by a second arrow, that this relieved the pain from the first.)

Central to the concepts of acupuncture is the idea of the body as self-healing, that it is a self-rectifying whole, a network of interrelating and interacting energies. Their even distribution and flow maintains health; any interruption, depletion or stagnation leads to disease. When this happens, acupuncture tries to aid these natural processes, helping the body to correct itself by a realignment or redirection of energy which the Chinese call Qi (pronounced 'chi').

So what is Qi? It is often translated as breath, life-force, vitality – or simply as that which makes us alive. If there is no Qi, there is no life. Strong and energetic people have plenty of Qi; tired and depressed people lack Qi. Along with the notion of Qi, acupuncture recognises a subtle energy system by which Qi is circulated through the body in a network of channels or 'meridians' along which lie the acupuncture points. When the acupuncture needle is inserted, it is the Qi that is affected. In some ways it is similar to the blood circulation and nervous system, but it is invisible to the eye.

Accepting this understanding of the body as an energetic and vibrating whole leads to a new approach to health and disease. It draws together all the diverse signs and symptoms of ill health to form a 'pattern of disharmony' which includes the mental/emotional state as much as physical problems. Yet it is not a system of medicine in isolation: it should be seen as one major method of treatment within a complete system that has a different perspective on health from that of orthodox Western medicine. The idea of treating a patient's headaches in one medical department, their period pains in another and their insomnia in a third would seem to them to be extraordinary since they believe there must be a common root.

Nowadays, there are two versions of acupuncture: one that

is traditional and combines it with herbal therapy, and one that is scientific and Westernised. The second rejects the existence of channels or 'meridians' and believes that acupuncture works via the nervous system, and that its effects can, in principle, be explained in terms of anatomy and physiology. There is as yet nothing to suggest that there is a great deal of difference between the two approaches in terms of results.

You will need to decide whether you are going to consult a lay practitioner (someone who may have had no formal training and possesses no accepted academic qualifications), or a doctor who is fully qualified through conventional medical training and who has undergone further training in acupuncture.

There are 1,800 lay practitioners affiliated to the British Acupuncture Council and 1,700 doctors who are members of the British Medical Acupuncture Society. The latter is a nationwide group of family doctors and hospital specialists who practise acupuncture alongside orthodox medicine. (See Useful Addresses on page 148).

The consultation

A considerable amount of time will be spent asking for details about your general condition. These questions can relate to all your physical, emotional and energetic signs and symptoms, and although some of them may appear unrelated, all can help the acupuncturist to form a more complete picture of your condition.

The practitioner will also ask to see your tongue. This is a very important source of information for the acupuncturist: the shape, colour, coating and texture of the various parts of your tongue yield information about the state of your organs. A healthy tongue should be reddish in colour with little or no fur, it should not appear swollen or contracted, neither should there be cracks on the surface or 'teeth marks' along the sides.

During the consultation, a full medical history is taken. Other important questions concern sensations of heat and cold; perspiration and whether this occurs during the day or night; headaches; again when they occur and in what part of the head; urination and defecation; including frequency of bladder movements, and any tendency to constipation or diarrhoea. Diet and sleep patterns are also relevant.

As a woman, you will be asked about your menstrual cycles, in particular their length, duration and heaviness of bleeding and whether there is pain and discomfort.

According to traditional Chinese medicine there are several different causes of heavy bleeding, and there may be a combination of causes in one woman. For example, the heavy bleeding may be diagnosed as 'hot blood' where the symptoms are very red, gushing blood, hot flushes and skin problems. Another diagnosis may be 'weak Qi' where the symptoms are fatigue and paler, dribbling blood.

You will be asked to undress, except for your underclothes, for the last part of the consultation. The acupuncturist will be touching any areas of your body that are painful, to feel for heat, cold, swelling, tightness or lack of skin tone. Specific acupuncture points may be touched to see if they are painful, particularly points on your abdomen and either side of your spine.

You may be surprised to see that the acupuncturist will take your pulse at both wrists and in three positions, by the index, middle and ring finger. Acupuncturists believe that they can assess the balance of energy from these three positions and gain the key to your internal state. Your pulses will be checked at intervals during treatment to monitor the energy changes.

Having gathered all this information, the acupuncturist formulates the appropriate treatment for you. The choice of acupuncture points differs with each patient; some may be used repeatedly until a particular imbalance is corrected.

Treatment

Some patients show very little sensitivity to the needles and do not feel anything when they are inserted. Others may be aware of increased sensitivity in particular areas or on particular meridians. In general, however, treatment should not be painful and when needle sensation occurs it should not last more than a few seconds. It can be described as a 'tingling' or a feeling of numbness radiating from the needle.

All registered acupuncturists are required by law to sterilise needles. Before undergoing any treatment, you should ask about the sterilisation procedures in use at the clinic. Disposable needles are available if you prefer, though they are more expensive.

Treatment might be once a week to begin with, then at longer intervals as the condition responds. It depends on you and your 'pattern of disharmony'. The average number of treatments is five.

> *After my treatments, my periods went from 18–20 to 26 days, my PMS was far less, and I felt well all over. Unfortunately, I am now going to have a hysterectomy because I have a retroverted uterus which is stuck to my bowel and is causing problems.* Jennifer (Derby)

Informing your GP

GPs responded in various ways when some of my respondents told them they were seeing an accupuncturist, ranging from, 'He thought it was a great idea . . .', 'The acupuncturist was recommended by my GP . . .', 'He was very encouraging and is now extremely pleased that I am better', to 'My GP is not interested . . .', 'He knows but is very sceptical'. By far the greater number were reluctant to tell their GPs.

How acupuncture works

Acupuncture stimulates the fine network of nerves running in the skin and sometimes nerves in the deeper tissues too. These then affect the central nervous system, blocking pain and altering the nervous system's control of other bodily organs. It is demonstrably untrue to say that the results of acupuncture are 'all in the mind'. After all, treatments have been success-fully carried out on very small children and animals. It is very unlikely that a cow could be hypnotised into health by a veterinary surgeon!

Case Study (1)

Elke, age 33. Married with one child. Occupation: Freelance translator

Seven years ago, Elke found she was bleeding in the middle of her menstrual cycle and that her period pains were severe.

'I had been on hormone tablets when I was 21 and these had regularised my periods, they became normal, so I was really worried about this change.'

She was treated for erosion of her cervix and had a laparoscopy and D & C the following year. But the heavy bleeding continued, various tablets were tried and once again she found herself on hormone tablets.

'Without them, I could not stand up during the first day of my period. The pain was so extreme, the blood loss so heavy that I rarely dared to leave the house. But I had to face the possibility of taking these tablets for years or having a hysterectomy – and I was not at all happy about either of those alternatives.

'A friend mentioned acupuncture and I thought – well why not? After four treatments, one a week between two periods, I felt like a normal person again: my periods were normal, the pain had gone – and so had the PMT. I now have treatment once a month, but this will probably be once every two months very soon and afterwards even less frequently.'

Case Study (2)

Caroline, age 49. Married with four children. Occupation: Regional Assistant Manager of company

'I began menstruating when I was ten years old and never had any problems with my periods. Then, when I was 46, my periods suddenly became much heavier for six months with mid-cycle bleeding. The doctor diagnosed a fibroid and an ultrasound scan revealed that it was over 5 centimetres/ 2 inches long. By this time I was experiencing some incontinence, so the doctor recommended a hysterectomy.

'The idea horrified me so I told the doctor that I wanted to try acupuncture first, and no objection was raised to this idea. I'd been interested in alternative therapies for a long time and had been to an acupuncturist for help with stress and tension.

'Where I think I am very fortunate is that complementary therapists practise in the same premises with my GP, so all I had to do was walk down the corridor and make an appointment with the acupuncturist.

'The mid-cycle bleeding stopped after two treatments and my periods normalised for about 18 months. Then the mid-cycle bleeding began again and further treatment alleviated 90 per cent of this. That happened at a time when I was going through a lot of stress at work which I'm sure did not help. As yet I have not had another scan but understand that fibroids shrink with the onset of the menopause.

'I am really pleased that I did not have a hysterectomy as I believe that not enough consideration is given to the "knock-on" effect of the removal of the uterus.'

Recent Research

In 1988, Dr Liu Wangcheng and his colleagues at the Heilongjiang Academy of Traditional Chinese Medicine in China treated 30 women with severe menstrual bleeding. Their average age was 36. All of them had suffered menstrual disorders for more than three months: menstruation had persisted for 9–15 days in 12 cases, for 16–30 days in 13 cases and over 30 days in five. Other possible causes of uterine bleeding, such as blood or liver disease, hypertension, gynaecological inflammation, tumours, injuries or foreign bodies (including intra-uterine devices) were ruled out.

Differentiation of syndromes

1. *Stagnancy of liver*: shortened or irregular menstrual cycles, incessant menstrual discharge of dark purplish blood with copious blood clots, distending pain and tenderness in the lower abdomen, bitterness in the mouth, depression, distending pain in the breasts, purple tongue or purple

dots on the tongue with scanty coating, and string-taut pulse.

2. *Deficiency in both heart and spleen*: prolonged or irregular menstrual cycles with menstrual discharge of pale red blood, sometimes more and sometimes less, dizziness, palpitations, insomnia, heat sensations in the chest, palms and soles, weakness of the limbs, sallow complexion, pale tongue with redder tip and borders, thin tongue coating and thready weak pulse.

3. *Deficiency in spleen*: prolonged menstrual cycles, excessive menstrual discharge of pale red blood with no or small clots, pale complexion, weakness of the limbs, anorexia, pale, plump and flabby tongue with 'teeth prints' at the borders, thin whitish tongue coating, deep thready pulse.

4. *Deficiency of liver and kidney*: shortened menstrual cycles, incessant menstrual discharge of bright red and sticky blood, sometimes more and sometimes less, aching and limpness in limbs, heat sensation in the chest, palms and soles, reddened tip and borders of the tongue with scanty coating, thready rapid pulse.

The procedure of the treatment consisted of (a) arresting the bleeding and (b) improving the general condition and regulating the menstrual cycles. Acupuncture was performed once daily with 15 days as a course. There was a three-day interval between courses.

Results of treatment

Bleeding stopped within seven days in 24 women and on the 7th–10th day in four women, but it continued or recurred in two cases.

Twenty cases were followed up for three menstrual cycles: bleeding was stopped and symptoms relieved within seven days of treatment in 16 cases, bleeding stopped within ten days of treatment in two cases but it was not stopped or recurred afterwards in the remaining two cases.

These results show that acupuncture was used successfully in treating 90 per cent of the women.

Medical Herbalism

I have suffered painful and irregular periods since I was 12 years old. Four years ago a hysterectomy was suggested which I did not believe to be the answer. I went to a medical herbalist and it has been so successful for me that if my two daughters have any trouble, I shall immediately take them to Mr H. Katrina (Leeds)

There can be little doubt that plants were the first source of medicines, and the use of herbs as a source of healing remedies is inherent in all cultures in all historical times. Experience showed primitive man which particular leaves could salve the wound of an arrow, and which could be boiled to cure a fever. Evidence that the poppy was used to relieve sickness and pain has been found in some early cave dwellings, where its seed was probably used for its soporific effects.

Over the centuries, plants have been sampled for food or patiently experimented with in an effort to find out more about their medicinal use. Who, for example, discovered that a tincture of opium from the poppy would stop children's crying, or that the oil from the beans of the castor tree, in small amounts, made a reliable purgative, while two or three of the beans themselves would prove fatal within a few hours? Or that the extracted oil would bring relief when applied to burns and septic wounds, besides making a useful fuel for lamps? Yet both these plants must have been regularly used for these purposes as some of their seed has been found in the ancient tombs of Egypt dated 1500BC. How many succumbed to the more virulent uses of these plants before the proper dose was found will never be known, but it was probably thousands.

So important did this information become to the community that it was committed to a caste of priest/physicians. Medicine became associated with magic, religion and astrology, although in 460BC the Hippocratic School attempted to separate herbal medicine from the occult and relate it to careful observation of the patient. It was Hippocrates who formulated the principle that treatment and dosage should be decided in accordance with the individual patient's requirement, and this is one of the cornerstones of modern-day medical herbalism, as is the belief that the whole plant should be prescribed.

These herbal remedies of antiquity became more accessible in the form of printed textbooks with the advent of printing during the Renaissance, but the dawn of scientific medicine in the seventeenth century with its emphasis on reason and experiment challenged these doctrines: the herbalists' ancient authority was further undermined by the emergence of inorganic remedies, and herbal remedies became almost obsolete.

However, in every rural community since pre-history there have probably been individuals, mostly women ('wise women') who were regarded as specialists in the art of using healing plants. They satisfied the needs of basic health care, treating injuries and illness and usually acting as midwives as well. Many of these women were tied to a larger network of 'women's culture' that handed down medical folklore, and this culture once embraced millions of women patients. It is this folk medicine of rural communities which, blended with traditional lore of the American Indians in North America in the eighteenth and nineteenth centuries, produced the patent medicines peddled by travelling 'medicine men', 'snake doctors' and 'quacks'. 'Quacks' is short for 'quacksalvers', people who applied salves of quicksilver (mercury).

Tainted with a reputation for superstition and quackery, coupled with the advances in medical science presided over by eminent doctors such as Pasteur, herbal practices were pushed into obscurity once more. The end of the last century saw a renewal of interest in medical herbalism, its practitioners treating people uneasy about the widespread use of drugs and their side-effects.

The consultation

The herbalist will give you a thorough examination and will need details of your medical history and eating lifestyle. Your blood pressure will be checked and the practitioner will be evaluating the overall balance of your body's systems –

musculo-skeletal, nervous, cardiovascular, digestive, genito-urinary and endocrine – to discover underlying and predisposing disharmonies.

It is you as a whole person who will be treated, not simply the complaint, so entirely different remedies may be prescribed to two patients apparently suffering from the same problems.

You are unlikely to need frequent consultations unless you have a condition which requires close monitoring and more regular examinations. You can simply telephone the herbalist when you need more medicine, and any adjustments can be made to the remedy if necessary.

Many patients note a measurable degree of improvement within the first month of treatment, but one to two months for every year of illness may be required if the condition is chronic.

I have suffered appallingly painful periods since I was 18. I was given drug treatment, then a laparoscopy which revealed that I had endometriosis. A hysterectomy was suggested but I was unhappy about this – I am a 24-year-old student and as yet have no children. There was a large improvement after starting herbal medicine and I can now eat normally during a pain-free period, continue studying and feel great! Vanessa (London)

Safety

It is a persistent and popular belief that herbs are safe and free from side-effects, but not all plants are safe. Many plants in Britain are known to be poisonous but few are dangerously so. However, the full effects of toxic constituents in plants are difficult to assess. Some such plants are known poisons, for example aconite, belladonna, mandrake, hemlock and white bryony. Under the terms of the Medicines Act 1968, herbal practitioners are permitted to use a few of these plants up to statutory maximum dosages, but these are not permitted for general sale.

The following are the herbs which would be considered:

- Helonias root
- Parsley
- Agnus castus
- Rosemary
- Blue cohosh (American)
- Beth root

- Shepherd's purse
- Lady's mantle
- White deadnettle
- Cramp bark
- Anemone pulsatilla
- Chamomile

A herbal remedy is usually a mixture of several herbs. Some herbalists grow at least a few of their stocks but usually they are bought commercially. Herbalists may use a mixture of British and European herbs, or add American and/or Chinese herbs if necessary. A few preparations rely on the use of fresh herbs, but the vast majority are dried specimens and, if stored well, they will last a long time, though not indefinitely.

Breaking down the herb samples to a suitable size used to be the hardest work of all the processes of preparation, entailing hours of labour with a pestle and mortar. Nowadays, the kitchen blender will perform many functions quite adequately.

Water or a mixture of water and ethyl alcohol is added. Sometimes acetic acid (vinegar), glycerol (or glycerine), ether and seed oils are used. A liquid is selected which will have the best chance of dissolving the required active ingredients. 'Woody' material, such as bark and roots, has to be infused in hot water for a certain period. Most herbal remedies are given in liquid form but capsules, pills, powders and lozenges can also be dispensed.

Combining medicines

Medical herbalists would not advise you to stop taking your drugs but would work alongside any orthodox treatment if deemed necessary. Many patients want to come off their prescribed drugs, and herbalists would aim to reduce or cease the need for them.

Until the age of 30 I could not arrange anything important around the time of my periods – exams were a nightmare and work was disrupted, in fact I had to turn down a promotion. I refused the gynaecologist's sugges-

tion of a hysterectomy, consulted a local herbalist and could not believe the difference after four weeks . . . Potential patients should not be discouraged if the treatment is slow to take effect. I actually felt worse before feeling better. Janice (Burnley)

Sensible measures

- Never persist with any herbal remedy after a moderate amount of time, preferably no more than several weeks, if it is not clearly improving your condition. Most herbs do not take months to work – it is the condition that sets the pace.
- Always challenge a treatment if, after four weeks, you think the herbal remedy is not useful or, even if there are doubts, stop the medicine for a time and see if it is still necessary.

Case Study (1)

Angela, age 43. Married with two children. Occupation: Charity shop manageress

'I can't remember a time when I wasn't on painkillers because my periods were so painful. There were always two days in the month when it was at its worst and I would sometimes pass out. I came to dread those days.

'Hormone tablets helped on and off for a couple of years but eventually I went to see a consultant who diagnosed endometriosis. He strongly recommended a hysterectomy as he told me it would only get worse. I was not happy with the idea of surgery and, remembering how a friend had been to a herbalist with beneficial results, decided to try this first. I actually felt quite encouraged as the consultant was not averse to the idea.

'There was little change in seven months, other than some slight lessening of pain, and then suddenly the pain and discomfort was minimal. My periods are now totally pain-free.'

Case Study (2)

Pat, age 53. Married with two children. Occupation: Antique dealer

'I'd been in and out of my doctor's surgery since I was 36 years old, trying every tablet and drug for period problems.

Some would work for a while, then all the symptoms of moodiness, irritability, pain, migraines, water retention and a very ugly swollen stomach would return. I had greasy hair and terrible facial spots so it's hardly surprising that I had long spells of depression.

'After a D & C I was just told it was 'messy' inside, nothing else. Then, a year later, a scan showed there were fibroids.

'I was told that hysterectomy was the answer but I hated the idea of this and was convinced there was another way. It was my doctor who suggested a herbalist.

'There was an improvement after one treatment and I continued with it regularly. My skin cleared and my hair became glossy and I felt so much better. All the symptoms were relieved and the quality of my life improved dramatically.

'Finding this herbalist was the best thing that has ever happened to me.'

Homoeopathy

Within the first month of homoeopathic treatment, there was an improvement in the monthly flooding and severe anaemia, and this has been maintained over the last two years. Jennifer (Bath)

I found it wonderful to be assessed by a practitioner who listened and noted all the symptoms. Annabel (Cardiff)

Nearly two hundred years ago, an eminent and conventionally qualified German physician published the first results of a form of treatment which he had developed and used experimentally on himself and his family. His name was Samuel Hahnemann, and he christened the principle of this treatment 'homoeopathy', from two Greek words meaning 'similar' and 'disease'.

It had all begun when he decided to see what might happen if he took some cinchona bark (which contains the drug now known as quinine). He was surprised to find he developed a fever and other symptoms associated with malaria. These symptoms then disappeared when he stopped taking the cinchona bark. Here was confirmation of Hippocrates' belief that if an individual who is suffering from an illness can be made to suffer symptoms similar to those produced by his illness, then he will be cured.

This 'like cures like' principle formed the basis of homoeopathy, but it was not the only one which distinguished Hahnemann's medical practice from that of his contemporaries. Dissatisfied with the medical practices of his day, which consisted mainly of 'bleeding' and the use of large doses of dangerous drugs, he decided to dispense smaller doses of medicine. To his surprise, he found that the more the remedy was diluted, the more active it became.

Orthodox medicine was unimpressed. This paradox – that less of a substance could be more acceptable – was, perhaps not surprisingly, unacceptable to the scientific thought of the time. Hahnemann and his followers were ridiculed, yet they continued to experiment with all sorts of things – salts, animal products and vegetable substances – collaborating in what he termed 'provings': over long periods they took small doses of various reputedly poisonous or medicinal substances, carefully noting the symptoms they produced. Patients suffering from similar symptoms were then treated with these substances with encouraging results.

An enormous amount of material was accumulated as the main source of knowledge about homoeopathy and, by the time he died in 1843, Hahnemann had done 'provings' on 99 substances. This increased to 600 more medicines by 1900, and today there are nearly 3,000 substances which are available to homoeopaths. The materials include onion, Indian hemp, honey-bee sting venom, snake venom and spiders, as well as sand, charcoal, common salt and pencil lead.

Hahnemann also advocated the use of single medicines rather than complex mixtures, reasoning that it was not possible to distinguish the effects of large numbers of drugs when they were mixed together.

In some ways, Hahnemann was a scientist, but in others he was a metaphysician or even a mystic. He believed life was sustained by a vital force and that disease was due to some outside influence which disturbed the smooth functioning of the vital force, thus inducing symptoms of illness – discover and remove the cause of the trouble, stimulate the vital healing force of nature and the patients would heal themselves.

As with acupuncture there are two versions of homoeopathy: one which lays great emphasis on the use of highly dilute medicines and on certain philosophical, even semi-mystical, ideas about disease and its causation, and a modern form which is based on fairly orthodox notions of pharmacology and largely ignores philosophical thought. But the essence of the homoeopathic principle remains the same, i.e. it is the patient who is treated rather than the disease.

The consultation

First of all, you need to decide whether you are going to consult a lay practitioner (someone who may have had no formal training and possesses no accepted academic qualifications), or a doctor who is fully qualified through conventional medical training and who has undergone further training in homoeopathy.

There are over 600 doctors in the Register of the Faculty of Homoeopathy, and it is estimated that in excess of 2,000 GPs are using some homoeopathy or referring to homoeopathic centres. There are five homoeopathic hospitals within the National Health Service – in London, Glasgow, Liverpool, Bristol and Tunbridge Wells – where patients are prescribed both orthodox medical treatment and homoeopathic remedies.

Your first appointment can last as long as two hours, as making the correct diagnosis is a vitally important part of the treatment. A lot will need to be known about you: your past health and life circumstances, the pattern of health in your family, your present condition – what are the particular symptoms? what makes them worse or better (warmth, cold, eating, drinking, moving about, lying down and so on . . .)? How do you feel about the condition (angry, resentful, depressed)? Your fears, moods and anxieties will be heard, so that a multidimensional picture of you as an individual emerges.

Referral

All responsible homoeopaths agree that many serious disorders – cancers, serious infections and so on – do need treatment from orthodox practitioners.

But assuming that you do not need to be referred, then the homoeopath will analyse all the information you have supplied and formulate the appropriate medicine.

You can obtain it from your pharmacist, both here and in European countries, and homoeopathic prescriptions are available under the National Health Service. Although they are completely different in their preparation and action, homoeopathic medicines look like any other medicines.

Safety

Homoeopathic remedies are completely safe, non-toxic and non-addictive.

Combining medicines

It is perfectly safe to take antibiotics with homoeopathic medicine, though the side-effects from the antibiotic may complicate the symptoms picture and make the choice of homoeopathic medicine more difficult.

There are a number of homoeopathic substances which have a very specific application in certain conditions, such as indigestion and bruising, and so they can successfully treat a large cross-section of the population. For instance, arnica ointment is very effective for healing bruises after an operation.

Some feeling of well-being should be experienced within one week, even though the symptoms remain. If this is entirely absent within two weeks of starting treatment, then an alternative medicine should be considered.

My doctor told me that a hysterectomy was the only solution for the prolapse of my womb. I decided to consult a homoeopath and have been taking the remedies for six months. I now have considerably more energy, am taking regular exercise such as horse riding, and I believe this has strengthened the muscles which hold my uterus in place, for I certainly have far less discomfort from the prolapse. Shirley (Wells)

Case Study (1)

Pamela, age 35. Single with one child. Occupation: Film librarian

'My problem started with ovulation pain which was very severe and sometimes lasted up to a week. I was already seeing a homoeopath and was given some treatment, but at the same time I was seeking some sort of diagnosis from the doctor for my own peace of mind. The doctor did not think the problem was gynaecological and things just got worse.

'Eventually I went to a Well Woman Clinic, the doctor examined me and told me straight away that I had an ovarian cyst. This was confirmed by laparoscopy. I had an operation to remove the cyst, using homoeopathic remedies before and afterwards to help recuperation.

'Endometriosis was found at the same time as the operation and hysterectomy was suggested as the long-term solution if the condition worsened. I was advised to go back on the Pill without a break to prevent ovulation, but didn't want to do this because I had given up the Pill after ten years because of side-effects.

'I am soon to have an ultrasound scan to see whether I have any more cysts as I still have pain on ovulation.

'On balance, I am glad I tried homoeopathy first as I felt improvement in my general well-being but I don't think it helped to reduce the size of the cyst or the severity of the symptoms overall. I think it is very important to think for yourself and not to accept things blindly, whether from orthodox or alternative practitioners.'

Recent research

Eighty-four women with various clinical manifestations of fibromyoma (fibroids) in the uterus received only homoeopathic treatment under the direction of Dr A Popov at the

Centre of Homoeopathy of the Ministry of Health of the Ukraine, Kiev, in the late 1980s.

The period of observation varied from one to three years. Pelvic examination was carried out every three months and ultrasound scanning every six months. In the course of these investigations, structure and volume of the tumour, size and localisation of the fibromatous nodes and the state of the endometrium were defined.

Results of treatment

Before treatment, pain was reported by 38 patients – this improved with treatment in 30 cases. Abnormal endometrial bleeding was observed in 40 women – this improved with treatment in 30 cases.

In 18 patients, while menorrhagia improved, further growth of the tumour was observed. On the other hand, nine women showed a decrease in myoma volume while endometrial bleeding did not improve. So, in women who had fibromyomata with abnormal endometrial bleeding, an inverse relationship was noted between tumour size and degree of menorrhagia.

It was concluded that homoeopathy could be a sufficiently effective method of treatment for patients with fibromyoma of the uterus, and that the optimum effects were achieved with small tumours.

It would be easy to conclude that there is a powerful placebo effect at work, and this attitude is encouraged by the shortage of reliable, responsible research in the field of alternative medicine in the UK. This is hardly surprising, considering that complementary medicine researchers have to compete with applicants from conventional medicine for funds. But it is in sharp contrast to the USA where a National Centre for Complementary and Alternative Medicine (NCCAM) supports research to the tune of £50 million a year – although I feel bound to add I have found no evidence of research into treatment of uterine dysfunctional bleeding by complementary medicine.

Personal recommendation is one way of choosing a complementary practitioner, so talk to people you know who have tried alternative therapies, and ask how they felt about the treatment they received. What did they think of the practitioner? Was the therapy being practised in clean and properly equipped premises? How much did the treatment cost, and how often did they receive it? Nowadays, reputable practitioners who advertise in the Yellow Pages include data about their professional organisations – if not you should check this when you make an appointment.

There are now more complementary practitioners than GPs in the UK and many offer time, a sympathetic manner and therapies which are concerned with the 'whole woman'. However, this is not always so and if, after an initial visit, you feel uncomfortable with your practitioner, then trust your judgement and do not continue.

Chapter Three

Hormone Replacement Therapy (HRT)

Hormones were first used on humans in the 1920s when they were extracted from sheep's dried ovaries. Ten years later the hormone oestrogen was being prescribed for women in the United States for menopausal 'complaints'. By the mid-1960s oestrogen therapy was hailed as the 'pathway to eternal youth' which would protect women from the 'living decay' of their middle years: skin wrinkles, middle-aged spread and sagging breasts would be eradicated along with crying spells, violent mood swings, aching joints and loss of memory. Replacing this would be eternally feminine, sexually active menopausal women with glowing skin and glossy hair. Sales of oestrogen supplements rocketed for throughout history women have tried to prevent the physical changes that occur with ageing.

Enthusiasm waned when medical research showed that women who took oestrogen were about five to fourteen times more likely to develop cancer of the endometrium of the uterus than those who were not taking oestrogen. This led to the addition of progestogen (a synthetic form of the hormone progesterone) which reduces the risk of endometrial cancer.

To date, HRT has failed to make the same impact in the UK as it has in the United States, in spite of years of scientific research and publicity which show that while properly prescribed HRT does not delay the changes of advancing years, it can help women to look and feel well and healthy.

Few areas of women's health stir up as much confusion and

debate as HRT. An understanding of what this debate is about should help you decide whether it is an appropriate therapy for you, as it may be recommended after hysterectomy.

What Are Hormones?

Hormones are chemical substances in your bloodstream and they circulate around your body playing an important part in sexual maturation, sexual arousal and the physical changes that go with it, and in reproduction. Their fluctuating levels will vary throughout your life, influencing your moods, activities and sensitivity as they constantly ebb and flow. Your hormonal make-up is as individual to you as your fingerprints.

Hormones also have an even more basic role: working with your nervous system, they link up different parts of your body, co-ordinating it into a whole distinct person and not just a set of disconnected organs.

Hormones are secreted by your *endocrine glands*, some of which are simply just a few cells, and others, like your *pituitary* (at the base of your brain) and your *thyroid* (in your neck) which are clearly visible without a microscope. Your thyroid gland affects every cell in your body, while growth hormone was needed when your height suddenly increased during puberty (any time from the age of nine).

Female Hormones

Of especial importance to you as a woman are your ovarian hormones – oestrogen and progesterone. Your body began producing oestrogen when you were a foetus of 15 to 20 weeks in your mother's womb, and it has played a major role in your body's change from that of a child to that of a mature woman.

You may have marvelled at the exquisitely soft skin of a baby. This is due to oestrogen, which causes an extra layer of fat to develop and so makes the skin ultra soft. By puberty, the level of oestrogen increases dramatically, changing the distribution of body fat so that you acquire the rounded contours of your feminine hips and thighs – this is often described as 'puppy fat'.

Certainly the word 'hormone' is an accurate one. It comes from the Greek word *horman* and it means 'to stir up or arouse to activity'. Maybe you can remember some of your emotions during puberty and adolescence – one day feeling elated, raring to go, and the next apathetic and unhappy. This is hardly surprising, given such bewildering and intricate changes.

It was the onset of menstruation (your monthly periods), usually some two years after this growth 'spurt', which signalled your preparation as a sexually active young woman and potential child-bearer, as your vagina, uterus and Fallopian tubes increased in size and your two ovaries began to develop ova (eggs).

Understanding your Ovaries

Your ovaries are egg-producing factories. If one ovary is not working, the other takes over its function. Oestrogen is secreted by the ovaries and this has a specific action on your genital system and breasts, as well as maintaining the health of your skin, mucous membranes and other body tissues.

Other hormones, such as progesterone and testosterone, are also produced by the ovaries. Progesterone thickens the lining of the womb in preparation for a fertilised egg. Testosterone helps to determine secondary sexual characteristics, such as hair growth and muscle mass, as well as increasing your sexual desire, activity and responsiveness.

Ovulation will slow down as you enter the menopause. This is a natural occurrence which signifies the completion of your life as a potential bearer of children. It can take up to five years to complete, and enormous changes take place in your body as it acquires a new balance with lower levels of hormones.

Your ovaries will continue to produce oestrogen, albeit at lower levels, for at least 12 years after the onset of a natural menopause, while testosterone is produced in the ovaries throughout your life.

Surgical removal of ovaries

One of the most common questions asked of hysterectomy contacts concerns the removal of ovaries at the time of hysterectomy, as Sarah of Winchester queried:

> *I'm 48 years old and I've had years of coping with heavy periods. I've tried everything, and the only answer is a hysterectomy. But my consultant says I should have my ovaries out at the same time because of the risk of ovarian cancer. I don't want them removed – what should I do?*

There is considerable controversy about this subject, and every woman in a similar situation needs to weigh the *risks* of developing ovarian cancer against the *benefits* of continued ovarian function. The latest research in Denmark, Japan and Australia, as well as that undertaken by the Cancer Research Campaign, indicates the following:

- 90 per cent of ovarian cancers occur in women after the age of 48 and those in their 50s and 60s are most at risk.
- Further risk factors include infertility, a well-documented family history of ovarian cancer, late menopause and lack of child-bearing.
- Oral contraception is associated with up to 70 per cent reduction in risk after ten or more years of use compared with never-use.
- Sterilisation reduces the risk of ovarian cancer by 39 per cent.
- Hysterectomy reduces the risk of ovarian cancer by 36 per cent (although the Danish nationwide controlled follow-up study of ovarian cancer after hysterectomy [1997] suggested this protection might fade out with time).
- Women preserving at least one ovary have a significantly decreased risk of ovarian cancer for at least ten years after the operation compared with women without hysterectomy.
- Women who had heavy periods before hysterectomy tended to have a lower risk of ovarian cancer after surgery than women who had average or light periods.

Once a decision has been reached, a letter to the consultant confirming it is strongly advised – in this way there can be no misunderstanding about this very important matter.

Hormone Replacement Therapy (HRT)

HRT is a course of the female hormones, oestrogen and progesterone, and it is prescribed if you need an artificial dose of hormones when the natural sources are inadequate. HRT can be recommended for the following reasons:

1. *To increase the supply of hormones at the time of your menopause*

There are about 10 million post-menopausal women in Britain, of whom approximately 75 per cent experience some of the following symptoms during their 'change':

● Hot flushes
● Mood changes
● Aches and pains in muscles and joints
● Dry vagina and discomfort with intercourse
● Night sweats and disturbed sleep
● Concentration and memory lapses
● Bladder irritability
● Dry hair and skin

2. *As the consequences of surgery involving the reproductive organs*

These could be:

● If you are a young woman having your uterus and ovaries removed: without HRT you are more likely to experience very severe menopausal symptoms.
● If you are a young woman and have had your ovaries removed: you have experienced an artificial menopause and without HRT you would be at greater risk of osteoporosis.
● If you are near to your menopause and your uterus is being removed but your ovaries retained: HRT could be recommended in view of potential menopausal symptoms.

- If you are near to your menopause and your uterus and ovaries are being removed: HRT would be strongly recommended.
- If you are near to your menopause, post-menopausal, disabled: HRT would be recommended, not only because of menopausal symptoms but because of the added difficulties of potential osteoporosis.

HRT is the only treatment which has been shown to prevent osteoporosis. This is a condition in which the bones become thinner and it is associated with a drop in the levels of oestrogen after the menopause. Women of Afro-Caribbean, Aboriginal and Mediterranean origin appear to be less susceptible than those who are white or Asian because they usually possess thicker bones and reach a greater bone mass at skeletal maturity.

> *One in every four white/Asian women has broken a wrist or hip bone or suffered a crush fracture of the spine by the age of 65 and half of all women have had a fracture by the age of 75.*

Women who are at greater risk of developing osteoporosis are:

- Women who are disabled
- Women who smoke
- Women who experience an early menopause whether natural or artificial
- Women who have a low body weight
- Women who are alcoholic

Widespread studies have established that the risk of death from coronary disease is reduced by half if you take HRT at a time (after the menopause) when your chances of having a heart attack increase sharply.

> **Your normal oestrogen level can be maintained if only half of one ovary remains after surgery.**

In 25 per cent of women who have had their wombs removed, the ovaries become less efficient and premature menopause sets in within two years. No one is quite certain why this happens but it could be due to a loss of blood supply to the ovaries, or because they become encased in thick adhesions following hysterectomy.

Is HRT suitable for all women?

No. Some women manufacture more oestrogen in their bodies than others do. Your oestrogen levels can be ascertained by having a blood test or a vaginal smear which will reveal the number of mature cells. Ask for a hormone test *before* having HRT, as you must know what your hormone level is normally.

There are a few medical reasons for not giving HRT, and it may not be suitable if you have a history of one of the following conditions:

- Endometriosis (unless it has been treated or has become quiescent post-menopausally)
- Breast cancer or cysts
- Cancer of the lining of the womb (the endometrium)
- Liver disease
- High blood pressure or if you have had a stroke
- A history of clotting of the deep leg veins or the lungs
- Any oestrogen dependent malignancy
- Untreated abnormal bleeding

Your doctor will need to examine you thoroughly, including checking your blood pressure, before starting the treatment, and then regularly afterwards when your prescription is renewed.

I have had no HRT as there is a family history of kidney failure and blood clots, so I rely on extra calcium, cod liver oil and evening primrose oil. Moira (Manchester)

What HRT treatment is available?

These are the main choices offered at the present time, all of which have different strengths:

1. Tablets

This is the most common form of HRT, and a number of different tablets are available.

If your uterus is intact, your tablets will contain both hormones, i.e. oestrogen and progesterone. If you took oestrogen on its own there would be a slightly greater than normal chance of your getting cancer of the uterus, so progesterone acts as a protective measure. You will experience some light bleeding but this is not the same as a period.

Sometimes the two hormones are combined in one tablet, sometimes they are taken separately.

If you have had a hysterectomy your uterus has been removed, therefore tablets containing only oestrogen will be prescribed.

2. A transdermal oestrogen patch (Estraderm)

This contains tiny doses of oestrogen which are released through the skin. You apply it to a small area below your waistline or your buttocks, where the movement of your body will not cause the skin to wrinkle. The patch will need to be changed twice a week.

3. Transdermal oestrogen and progesterone patches (Estracombi)

This is a combined patch for women who have their uteri. Prior to this, it was necessary for women using an oestrogen patch to supplement it with progestogen tablets. Each used patch should be removed after three to four days.

4. A hormone implant

The doctor (usually in a hospital) injects a little local anaesthetic into the skin of your abdomen. A tiny cut is then made and a pellet containing oestrogen is inserted through a tube. The tube is removed and the pellet pushed down into the fat under the skin. The opening is closed either with a stitch or a plaster. The hormones are slowly absorbed and can last up to nine months, according to the dose. This treatment is combined with progestogen tablets if you have your uterus.

5. Tibolone (Livial)

This is effective in reducing the severity and frequency of hot flushes and in relieving sweating and headaches in post-menopausal women who have an intact uterus. It is not recommended for use until one year after the cessation of menstruation.

6. Oestrogen cream

This is available when treatment is mainly required for symptoms such as vaginal dryness and dyspareunia (pain during intercourse) – very small doses applied with the fingers are often enough. But the absorption of oestrogen varies unpredictably and if symptoms occur when treatment is discontinued, then tablets may be suggested.

---

* REMEMBER *

IF YOU HAVE HAD A HYSTERECTOMY, YOU WILL NOT NEED
THE PROGESTERONE IN YOUR HRT.

What about side-effects?

- Some women feel nauseous and may vomit after taking hormone tablets. The strength of the dosage may need to be changed if this does not settle down after a couple of weeks.
- There may be wound infection at the site of an implant and it may not be absorbed.
- Your breasts may swell and become tender – again, this often wears off after a couple of weeks, but if not and it becomes a major problem, then you will need a different HRT preparation.
- Patches can cause a skin irritation and some women become fidgety and hyperactive after putting on their patches.
- If you have an implant and experience any side-effects it will be impossible to remove it, so you might have to wait several months before trying an alternative form of HRT, whereas a patch or tablet can be discontinued immediately. Oestrogen levels are higher than with other forms of HRT and this may not be beneficial. It also appears that in some women the body may become accustomed to continued high levels of oestrogen and produce symptoms characteristic of oestrogen deficiency when the levels are high but just beginning to fall. Consequently, further implants may be given too soon.

I was started on HRT in the form of tablets. These produced high blood pressure and headaches so I was changed to patches. They changed my life – the night sweats and flushes disappeared, as did my sore vagina. Annette (Brunei)

I was given an oestrogen implant, even though I requested patches. During the first month I experienced severe hot flushes, dizziness, palpitations and intense headaches. I am to have a patch when the implant stops working. Yvonne (Birmingham)

I have heard that HRT can cause breast cancer – is this true?

Most contention and uncertainty relate to HRT and the risk of breast cancer, and there is conflicting data. Some show that the risk is reduced whereas other data suggest a slight increase. What is certainly true is that some types of breast cancer are fast-growing and quickly fatal while others develop very slowly, over 18 to 20 years or even longer. We should all be concerned about this as it may be a long time before an effect is seen clinically. The issue is further complicated because breast tissue is influenced by changing levels of hormones – but there are also other factors which determine the development of this group of cancers, such as diet and heredity.

It is not correct to say that HRT can cause breast cancer but it may play a part in producing abnormal changes in the breast tissue which could lead to cancer.

Recent research

In January 2000, researchers at the National Cancer Institute in Rockville, Maryland, USA, released the results of a study of just under 45,000 post-menopausal women who took part in a breast cancer detection project between 1980–1995. It found that over 2,000 of the women had developed the disease. The findings listed here confirm the potential hazards and uncertainties in the use of HRT.

- The relative risk of developing breast cancer was 20 per cent higher for those who had taken HRT containing oestrogen than for women who had never taken HRT.
- The risk was 40 per cent higher for women who had taken oestrogen with progestogen.
- Thin women are more at risk if they take oestrogen alone.

It looks as though there are both risks and benefits – how can I come to a decision about it?

First, you need to determine whether you are experiencing symptoms associated with the menopause (see the chart below).

Please tick one box for each symptom

Symptoms	*Severe*		*Moderate*		*Mild*		*None*	
1. **Hot flushes**	12		8		4		0	
2. **Sweating attacks**	12		8		4		0	
3. **Tension/irritability**	3		2		1		0	
4. **Dryness of the vagina/irritation**	3		2		1		0	
5. **Loss of interest in sexual relations** (ignore if not applicable)	3		2		1		0	
6. **Insomnia**	3		2		1		0	
7. **Lack of energy**	3		2		1		0	
8. **Hair/skin changes**	3		2		1		0	
9. **Muscular and/or joint pains**	3		2		1		0	
10. **Changes in memory/concentration**	3		2		1		0	

Age: Under 45 ☐   45–49 ☐   50–54 ☐   Over 54 ☐

When complete, total all the scores. A score of 30 or more strongly suggests that symptoms are associated with the menopause, although a low score will not exclude this.

Now ask yourself the following:

How much are these symptoms affecting my life at present, bearing in mind that the menopause can last for up to five years?
HRT will alleviate some of the symptoms, especially the hot flushes and vaginal dryness.

Did both or either of my grandmothers, mother, aunts or older sisters suffer from osteoporosis? Did they become noticeably shorter or more stooped as they grew older?
HRT will protect against fractures of the wrist, spine and hip. If HRT is taken for at least five years at the time of the menopause, your risk of having a fracture in later life is halved.

Does my family history include many individuals with heart attacks and strokes?
HRT will protect against heart disease.

Thus in three major ways, HRT can be of positive benefit. But you now need to ask further questions:

Have I or any female member of my family experienced breast cysts or breast cancer?
HRT may produce abnormal tissue changes in your breasts which might lead to cancer.

How long might I need to take HRT?
One to six months might be sufficient if you want to alleviate menopausal symptoms alone. But if your natural menopause is early, or you have had your ovaries removed and undergone radiotherapy before the age of your menopause, then you will need HRT at least until the age of 50 and possibly for a further ten years.

Only you can really decide whether to go on to HRT. Your decision may be fairly clear-cut: you may have experienced a relatively trouble-free menopause but be concerned because your mother is showing the same indications of osteoporosis as her mother did. In this case you will obviously benefit from it. Or you may have had a hysterectomy in your early forties, retained your ovaries and lead a healthy, fit and active life during your menopause. You may decide to supplement your diet with Vitamin D and calcium, and maintain regular daily exercise, especially 'foot-to-ground' exercise like walking, jogging, running and playing tennis, rather than embark on the therapy.

Many women find themselves somewhere in the middle of these two situations and are still uncertain, even when they are taking HRT. The following extracts from letters to the hysterectomy contacts (listed under Useful Addresses on page 148) testify to the uncertainties about the subject.

I had a hysterectomy nine months ago for heavy bleeding and was given HRT. I was all right at first but now I'm getting so depressed. I'm up and down all the time, crying at the slightest little thing that goes wrong. Is this because of the HRT?
It might be. You need to discuss this with your GP or consultant. A different type of HRT could be suggested or an adjustment to the dose. You could also try going without it for a week and see if it makes any difference. Perhaps you also need to look at what is going on in your life at present: could there be personal worries or family problems that need to be sorted out?

How soon can I go on to HRT after my hysterectomy? And will I feel the effects straight away?
If HRT is recommended following your hysterectomy, you will be able to begin it almost immediately if the decision was made by you and your consultant. The effects, such as the control of hot flushes and vaginal dryness, will be felt within a week.

I was sweating so much at night, sometimes I had to change the sheets a couple of times, and I was very irritable. My doctor put me on HRT as he said it was the 'change'. It's better but I thought it would all go away and it hasn't. I'm still moody at times. Am I getting enough HRT? And how does the doctor know when it's the right amount?

HRT is sometimes a matter of 'trial and error' as there are several different types and strengths available. Your GP will adjust the type and/or dosage until your symptoms diminish. However, do not blame the 'change' for everything: take a look at other changes that might be going on at present – your children may be leaving home, or perhaps you suddenly have to face caring for an elderly parent or cope with unexpected redundancy at work.

I had a hysterectomy ten years ago but retained my ovaries. I have now started the menopause and want to go on HRT, especially as the sight of my mother crippled by osteoporosis is causing me such anguish, added to which a bone scan has revealed that my bone density is far lower than it should be. However, I have a history of breast cysts and the specialist is unhappy about my taking HRT. What would you advise?
Discuss your fears and anxieties with your GP and, if possible, with your specialist again. You could also request a second opinion. Gather all the information that you can and consider all the risks and benefits, then decide which option *you* feel presents the greater risk. If you decide to take HRT, make sure that you have regular checks and mammograms (breast X-rays). If you decide not to take HRT, you need to ensure that you are on a good diet with plenty of fresh fruit and vegetables, in addition to foods rich in calcium and Vitamin D, and that you are taking regular exercise.

The potential market for HRT is huge. It is increasingly discussed in the media, yet fewer than one woman in ten is taking it. One reason is a deep-seated resistance among doctors, many of whom are uninterested in the subject generally. And it is not so long ago – in 1970, to be precise – that the implications of oestrogen deficiency were poorly understood, as the following experience testifies.

I had a hysterectomy when I was 34 years old and after three months' convalescence, returned to work. Several weeks later I felt depressed – having always been a lively, bubbly person, I couldn't understand my lethargy . . .

The next three years were spent taking a variety of the magic anti-depressants . . . At my lowest ebb, something snapped and I overdosed on sleeping tablets. I was hospitalised, and the next day transferred to the local mental hospital. Over the three weeks that I was detained in that place, I was given a course of electric shock treatment. 'Horrified' does not begin to describe my feelings. I discharged myself and never went back.

One day, while waiting in my dentist's surgery, I was reading a magazine and came across the story of a woman who could have been myself, her history was a replica of mine. Somehow she had learned of HRT, it had saved her sanity . . . When I got home, I phoned the magazine, obtained the addresses of clinics carrying out the treatment, and made an appointment. Following tests and examinations, the consultant found that my ovaries were no longer producing oestrogen. I had also lost 5 centimetres/2 inches in height during the three years of illness. I was told that I had experienced a traumatic menopause immediately after the operation . . . Within four weeks of the HRT treatment I felt reborn! Adeline (Swindon)

There are justifiable concerns about a therapy which produces controversial data. But we need to recognise that, until the latter end of the 1800s, a woman's chance of living past the age of 45 was only 50/50. Modern medicine and improved nutrition have given us an average life expectancy of 75 years or more. This means that many of us can now hope to live about a third of our lives after the reproductive lifespan has finished.

While HRT is no substitute for a healthy lifestyle, it is a valuable insurance policy against arm and wrist fractures, back pain and a stooped, curved spine; it can be a helpful short-term treatment during the menopause, and it is strongly recommended if you have your ovaries removed surgically.

Having read about HRT, you may feel uneasy or unconvinced about the need to take it – or indeed, you may have a medical condition which precludes the treatment – so the following alternatives are suggested.

Self-help

If sexual intercourse and/or masturbation is part of your life and your vagina takes longer to lubricate or dries out quickly during and after arousal, use K-Y jelly which is sterile, greaseless, water soluble and non-irritating.

Hot flushes can be alleviated by:

- wearing several layers of clothing so that you can easily adapt to the most comfortable temperature;
- using cotton underwear rather than nylon which will only aggravate your discomfort during the sweats;
- sleeping on cotton sheets with lightweight blankets; if you have a duvet, check the contents. Synthetic fibres may increase your discomfort if you wake up drenched in sweat at night;
- buying some hand-held, battery-driven fans (from either Woolworths or Argos) and keeping them where they are readily available: by your bed, in the kitchen, in your handbag, etc. These will generate cooling air more quickly than an ordinary fan;
- limiting your intake of alcohol and coffee, both of which tend to encourage hot flushes. The more caffeine you put in your body, the more calcium you lose; the more alcohol you drink, the less calcium is absorbed.

Maintain a healthy eating lifestyle with plenty of fresh vegetables and fresh fruit every day. Try eating potatoes with their skins on, rather than peeling them – as well as the taste being so much better, your fibre intake will improve, as it will if you bake with wholemeal flour rather than white. Fibre is extremely important: it absorbs water and contributes to the growth of beneficial bacteria in your gut, thus making a bulky stool, providing exercise for your bowel and keeping your intestine in healthy working order.

After the menopause you should have 1500 mg of calcium every day: the table on page 90 shows you how to achieve this with a balanced intake of calcium-rich foods.

Ways of increasing calcium intake

Daily requirement		
	before menopause	1,000 mg
	after menopause	1,500 mg

Calcium content of pills available over the counter	*Pills providing 600 mg*
Calcium gluconate 600 mg contains 54 mg calcium	12
Calcium lactate 300 mg contains 44 mg calcium	14
Sandocal – 4.5 g contains 400 mg calcium	1^1/2

Calcium content of common foods in mg per 100 g (3^1/2 oz approx) of food

Dairy	mg
Cheese	
Cheddar	800
Cottage (low-fat soft cheese)	60
Danish blue	580
Edam	740
Parmesan	1,220
processed	700
spread	510
Cream	79
Egg (whole)	52
Egg (yolk)	130
Milk (98 ml/3.53 fl oz)	120
Yoghurt – low fat (145 ml/5 oz)	180

Vegetables	mg
Beans, haricot (navy)	180
kidney	140
Broccoli	100
Cabbage	53
Chick peas	140
Greens, turnip, kale, collard, mustard	98
Olives in brine	61
Parsley	330
Peas (boiled/frozen)	31
Spinach (boiled)	600
Spring onions	140
Watercress	220

Meat and fish	mg

Meat contains very small amounts of calcium, as does fish. Meat pies and fish in batter contain calcium in the flour. Canned pilchards and sardines, sprats and whitebait contain calcium in the bones.

Boiled prawns	150
Canned crab	120
pilchards	300
salmon	93
sardines	460–550
Fried sprats	620–710
whitebait	860
Fish paste	280
Steamed scallops	120

Fruit	mg
Apricots, dried	92
Blackcurrants, raw	60
Currants, dried	95
Figs, dried	280
Lemon, whole	110
Rhubarb, raw	100

Nuts (shelled weight)	mg
Almonds	250
Barcelonas	170
Brazils	180
Peanuts (groundnuts), roasted and salted	61
Sesame seeds	870

Drinks (dry weight)	mg
Cocoa powder	130
Coffee, ground	130
instant	160
Malted milk drink (Horlicks)	230
Tea, Indian	430

Cooking ingredients	mg
Curry powder	640
Mustard, dry	330
Pepper	130
Salt, block	230
Stock cubes (depending on brand)	180
Yeast, dried	80

Flour and baked foods	mg
Bread (white or brown)	100
Hovis (UK)	150
Cake, sponge (fatless)	140
rock (individual fruit cakes)	390
Flour, plain (cake)	130
self-raising	350
Soya flour	210–40
Wheat bran	110

Supplements such as evening primrose oil (which contains gamma-linolenic acid as well as phyto-oestrogens) and cod-liver oil help with the regulation and control of cell growth, blood pressure and the cardiovascular system (as well as the menstrual cycle).

Try to take plenty of exercise – walking, cycling or swimming. If you go running, wear first-class training shoes, otherwise the shock of impact might damage your weight-bearing joints.

You might also like to consider the Linda Kearns cake.

After 13 years on HRT, Linda decided to discontinue taking it but found her menopausal symptoms, such as hot flushes, returned. Always interested in an alternative approach to health, she began reading about oestrogens in plants. On discovering that these occur in soya products – linseeds, lentils, chickpeas, mung beans, sunflower, pumpkin and sesame seeds – she mixed some of these ingredients together in the form of a cake.

The recipe for this cake is on page 92. It is now being made by a bakery in Yorkshire and I have included Mail Order details. It is evidently a success, as upwards of 2,000 cakes are baked every day and sold throughout the United Kingdom.

Recipe for the Linda Kearns cake

Ingredients
100 g/4 oz soya flour
100 g/4 oz wholewheat flour
100 g/4 oz porridge oats
100 g/4 oz linseeds
50 g/2 oz sunflower seeds
50 g/2 oz pumpkin seeds
50 g/2 oz sesame seeds
50 g/2 oz flaked almonds
2 pieces of stem ginger, finely chopped
200 g/8 oz raisins
1/2 teaspoon nutmeg
1/2 teaspoon cinnamon
1/2 teaspoon ground ginger
Approx 900 ml/3/4 litre soya milk
1 tablespoon malt extract

Place the dry ingredients into a large bowl and mix thoroughly
– then add the soya milk and malt extract. Mix well and leave
to soak for about half an hour. If the mixture is too stiff, add
more soya milk. Spoon into 2 loaf tins lined with greaseproof
paper brushed with oil. Bake in the oven Gas Mark 5/190°C
for about 1 1/4 hours or until cooked through – test for this
with a skewer. Turn out and leave to cool. It is delicious with
butter or spread. Ideally, eat a slice a day.

> The Linda Kearns cake is *not* artificial HRT. It is a cake
> containing *only* the ingredients listed which themselves
> contain natural plant phyto-oestrogens.

The cake is available by Mail Order from Foster's Bakery,
Barnsley, Yorkshire. Tel: (01226) 381712

Chapter Four
Part 1
Time to Prepare

I got myself fit before the operation going on a diet, and I took a lot of regular exercise which helped with my recovery. Janet (London)

During the few weeks prior to the operation, I found I was able to express many of my feelings about being childless. Yvonne (Belfast)

Having made your decision, now is the time to start preparing for the operation, even if you do not have a definite date for admission to hospital. You may be given two or three weeks' notice; equally you may receive two or three days' notice if a bed becomes unexpectedly available. Now could be the time to consider the following questions:

Physical fitness

Am I reasonably fit and active? Do I enjoy any physical activity – walking the dog/cycling/swimming/exercise classes? Am I an acceptable weight?

If the answers are 'No', then now is the time to embark on a 'keep fit' regime – go swimming two or three times a week, join an aerobics class. Your rate of recovery post-operatively will be improved if your body is in good shape.

Am I overweight? If so, now is the time to try and shed some of the excess – even a few pounds will make a difference, both to your physical appearance and to your morale.

Do I smoke? Could this be the opportunity for me to kick the habit? (If not, at least try to cut down for a week before the operation so that you are in the best possible condition for the anaesthetic). And remember – nowadays many hospitals do not have a smoking room, so smoking afterwards may be impossible.

Taking Vitamins C, B and E is recommended as a way of building yourself up before going into hospital, as is a two-day grape fast during which only grapes are eaten and unsweetened grape juice and bottled water drunk – this purifies the blood stream, cleaning out waste products and sharpening the mind.

Emotional well-being

Have I made the right decision? Am I worried about any particular issues? If so, do I need to talk about them now?

It is very important to talk about your feelings with your partner, if you have one – and for you to listen to your partner's feelings. These can range from great relief – an end is in sight to the frequent disruption, distress and exhaustion – to great sadness if you will now either never have a child or your son/daughter will never have a brother or sister. You may have a new partner and assumed that at some time a baby would be part of your relationship. All sorts of feelings can surface in this time of shock and grief, even the wider implications that maybe your partner's parents or yours will never become grandparents.

For you, hysterectomy may be followed by further treatment such as radiotherapy, and the prospect of this can seem daunting.

You may feel shocked at the impending loss of your womb, seeing it as not only an important part of your body but your very 'womanhood', frightened that somehow you will be less of a woman, that it will affect your sexuality.

If it is difficult to make sense of all these feelings, and if it is becoming confused and muddled, as a first step write down the following and add a word from those in the brackets:

I feel . . . (unhappy/shocked/sad/angry/frightened/guilty/miserable/worried /confused/embarrassed) because . . .

and describe what you are feeling. For instance, you might write the following:

'I feel frightened because sex won't be the same.'

or

'I feel worried because I might be depressed like I was after the children were born.'

Show this to your partner, explain that you need to talk about it, and fix a time when you can be together on your own without interruption. If you share these fears (recognising that both of you are scared and need to understand what is going to happen) and look for the answers either in this book, by talking to your doctor, or telephoning one of the hysterectomy contacts (see Useful Addresses, page 148), then your anxieties will lessen.

Perhaps your partner also needs to clarify some worries and will be able to write *'I feel . . . because . . .'* – so that this concern can be shared and resolved in a similar way.

Not all partners are able to respond in such a positive way. It may be embarrassing or difficult to discuss, so talking to other women who have had a hysterectomy can be helpful.

Domestic arrangements

How will they manage without me? And what about when I get home – who is going to help?

Worrying about what is/is not happening at home is not ideal when you are in hospital. This is where partners, family and friends can be involved.

Accept offers of all help, both for when you are in hospital and when you are home.

Write the offers down on a wall calendar and make sure that all your family know where this is.

If you have children, they will need to know about your intended absence, how long you might be in hospital and whether they can visit you. The actual explanation will depend on their ages: very young children need to feel reassured you are coming home, as well as secure in the consistent care of another adult, preferably one already known to them.

Plan ahead for your return home: once you begin to feel stronger, time may hang heavily if you are used to an active life. Interests and hobbies which you can pick up and put down when you feel tired are ideal – craft work such as knitting, sewing and tapestry, or jigsaw puzzles, crosswords, and books and magazines to read.

> *Before I went into hospital I gathered up shoe boxes full of photographs going back some 20 years, then when I was convalescing, sorted all of them into albums. It was very therapeutic.* Muriel (Stafford)

> *I had plenty of time to plan the children's summer holidays, find an au pair, stock the freezer, give up the Pill, alcohol, and have a good, healthy holiday.* Grace (Croydon)

Sick pay and benefits

If you work for an employer and earn enough money to pay Class 1 National Insurance (NI) contributions (including married women's reduced rate contributions) you will usually get Statutory Sick Pay (SSP) when you are off sick for four days in a row. SSP is paid to you by your employer for up to 28 weeks in a spell of sickness. (Further information is in Leaflet NI245 available from the Benefits Agency.)

Are you a member of a union? If so, find out what benefits are payable – convalescence might be one of them.

If, however, you are not in paid employment at present, and have chosen to put your energies into your family and home, then you will not be eligible even for Sickness Benefit unless you have paid enough appropriate NI contributions for two complete tax years before making a claim. Any NI contributions you may have made while in former paid employment are completely disregarded.

Going it Alone

Perhaps you are single, divorced or widowed, and any children are now independent and living away. Positive planning is needed.

- Telephone a hysterectomy contact (see Useful Addresses on p. 148). You will be able to talk about your concerns and establish a supportive link. There might also be an opportunity to meet other women in a similar situation.
- Alternatively, there may be meetings concerned with individual health issues at your GP's surgery, and Well Women Centres offer a service which covers all aspects of women's physical and emotional well-being including counselling services.
- If you are paid SSP, could it be used to pay for a home help, at least for the first four weeks?
- You may be eligible for Incapacity Benefit, so contact your nearest social security office for a claim form.
- Climbing up and down stairs will be exhausting for the first few days, as well as potentially dangerous if you fall. You might feel more comfortable if you were able to sleep downstairs.
- Have you got easy access to your kitchen? You will not be able to lift a kettle full of water – the answer is to put cups of water in the kettle or to use a lightweight plastic jug.
- Stock up with enough frozen/canned/instant food for at least a week, especially if access to shops is normally difficult for you.
- If you own a dog, you will need to make arrangements for its care for at least four weeks after your return home.

I'm a single Mum of 39 with a son of 12, and I put off having the operation even though I was in agony because I was so frightened I might die, and then he'd be on his own. Someone put me in touch with a hysterectomy contact – I talked and talked, and got a lot sorted. That's why the op went OK. Liz (Oxford)

'Going it alone' has one advantage – you have only yourself to consider. Once the first few weeks of transitory discomfort have passed you can recover at your own pace without the pressures of family life. Friends and neighbours can ease the lonely times, as can maintaining the contacts made in hospital – indeed, many long-lasting friendships arise out of this common experience of adversity.

One day, you will receive a letter advising you of the date of your admission to hospital together with a list of things to take with you, such as night clothes – 'shortie' nightdresses with a front opening and made of cotton are better than nylon ones, which can become uncomfortable in a warm hospital – toiletries and 10 and 20 pence coins for the payphone.

There may also be an invitation to visit the ward beforehand so that you can familiarise yourself with the surroundings and meet the nursing staff.

I filled my case with goodies – hand cream, nail file, pretty new nighties, a romantic book of Catherine Cookson's, talc and a fluffy pink towel. I had my hair cut, styled and highlighted – this was a great booster, adding confidence before and after the op. Gina (Edgware)

I'd advise anyone going into hospital to take their own supply of soft medicines such as relief for indigestion and constipation. Monica (East Grinstead)

Chapter Four
Part 2
Hospital

The first GP I saw and subsequent hospital doctors all discussed the removal of my womb in much the same way that they might have talked about an appendectomy or even the removal of an ingrowing toenail. AND IT IS NOT THE SAME! Christine (London)

One lady I met thought that her operation would mean one night in hospital and work the next week! Dale (Isle of Wight)

Each hospital has its own routine and admission procedure and you will usually be admitted a day before the operation. It is very seldom that a hysterectomy is performed on the day of admission, unless it is a most severe and acute emergency.

Once you have been admitted, you will be shown to your bed in the ward. The nurse will ask you to change into your night clothes, and get into bed, which may well seem a little strange if it is in the middle of the afternoon! But it is another sign that you are now dependent on others to tell you what to do, when and how, as you cross from being an 'outsider' to an 'in-patient'.

The ward will become familiar to you during this time of rest and relaxation, as you observe the daily 'comings and goings' of patients and medical personnel. If you are in an open ward, get to know your neighbours, as mutual support and encouragement will help all of you post-operatively.

Routine Preparation

At some stage in the day you will be given a thorough examination by the SENIOR HOUSE OFFICER, who will want to know the following:

- Your past medical history
- If you are taking any medication of any kind
- If you are allergic to anything
- If you have a special diet.

The procedure of the operation will be discussed with you, and if you have any questions, doubts or fears, do talk about them, even if you think they might seem trivial – you will recover far more quickly if you understand what is being done to you.

You will be asked to read and sign a consent form – again, query anything that is not clear on the form. Your consent to the operation is required by law.

THE NURSING STAFF will carry out the following investigations:

- You will be weighed to determine the amount of anaesthetic needed.
- Your blood pressure and pulse will be checked.
- A sample of your blood will be taken for analysis, in case you need a blood transfusion.
- A urine sample will be taken so that any infections or irregularities can be checked.
- If you have any heart problems, or are over the age of 50, an ECG (an electrocardiograph, which is a tracing of your heart) will be taken.

If you are a patient in a teaching hospital, some of these routine tasks and interviews can be carried out by medical students. As a patient, you have the right to refuse student examinations.

You may see your consultant gynaecologist who will be performing the operation, and you will certainly be visited by the anaesthetist and physiotherapist.

The Anaesthetist

The anaesthetist checks that your lungs and chest are clear so that there will be no trouble from bronchitis or any other chest infection. If you are worried about anaesthesia, or have had a bad reaction to it previously, then now is the chance to discuss your fears. Sometimes an epidural anaesthetic is used – this is an injection of anaesthetic into the outer lining of the spinal cord – and the patient remains conscious throughout the operation.

I was sick for a very long time after previous anaesthetics, so I was worried about being ill as well as coping post-operatively. I asked for an epidural, and all the implications were discussed. Although initially reluctant, the anaesthetist eventually agreed to it. Caroline (Bristol)

Implications of an epidural

- A calm temperament is essential as, once the epidural is administered, you will wait half an hour in the recovery room, so that it can take full effect. During this time, there will be other patients who are recovering, some of whom may sound disturbed.
- You need to be able to withstand pain, as 100 per cent pain relief cannot be guaranteed for the entire operation.
- A contingency plan should be agreed between you and the anaesthetist, just in case you find it unbearable.

I found it totally acceptable. Afterwards, the anaesthetist told me it was the first time both he and the consultant had performed a hysterectomy using an epidural. Although I am glad I did not know this before the operation, on reflection my admiration for them increased – they had listened to me and had accepted my request, however apprehensive they might have been. Caroline (Bristol)

The Physiotherapist

The physiotherapist will explain the importance of regaining mobility as soon as possible so that your blood starts circulating normally, thus avoiding any potential blood clotting. You will be shown the following:

Deep breathing exercises This type of breathing will ensure a good supply of oxygen to your lungs and help to reduce the effect of the anaesthetic.

Leg exercises These start with simple ankle movements and curling and stretching your toes, and progress to exercises which you can continue once you are home. Previously simple movements, such as getting in and out of bed, are difficult after this major operation, and even turning over in bed, sitting up and changing positions can be painful. You may see other women in the ward struggling with all of this after their operations.

Now is a good time to practise the following way of getting out of bed from a lying position:

Take a deep breath in to the bottom of your lungs and release it slowly as you

- bend your knees upwards
- roll on to your side, bringing your arms across your bust to the side of the bed
- at the same time as your legs swing down towards the floor, push against your bed with the elbow of one arm and the hand of the other arm. Ease yourself into a sitting position.
- Do all this in reverse to get into bed again.

Your preparation is now nearly complete. But you may wonder what it will be like when you wake up . . . you may have heard the words 'drip' and 'catheter' without really knowing what they mean – and patients are very seldom warned in advance, so suddenly being aware of various tubes attached to your body might be alarming.

Neither my husband or I had ever seen anyone immedi-
ately after an operation, and we did not know there
would be a drip, a drainage tube and a catheter. When
my husband and our daughter first came to see me, she
nearly fainted at the sight, and a year later told me that
she thought I was dying. Isobel (London)

A drip

An intravenous infusion of salt and sugar (passing from a bag
into a vein, usually in your arm) will be in action immediately following surgery. This replaces the fluid you normally take
by mouth, as the anaesthetic will stop the normal function of
the gut for a while, and, until it returns to normal, you will be
asked not to drink. If you do so, you will be sick. The drip will
be kept in position for between 24 and 48 hours after your
operation.

A drainage tube

After surgery, excess fluid is produced at the operation site. To
prevent it accumulating under the wound, a drainage tube
may be attached by the surgeon and this will channel the fluid
into a bottle. It will be removed in two or three days when
drainage stops. It is not usually painful but may be uncomfortable.

A catheter

A catheter is a plastic tube passed up the urethra (the water
pipe in front of the entrance to the vagina) to drain the bladder and keep it empty, and it will be inserted while you are
unconscious in theatre to ensure that your bladder is empty
before the operation begins.

Sometimes, the catheter is left in the bladder, especially
after vaginal hysterectomy, so that the discomfort of using
bedpans in the immediate post-operative period is avoided.
The end of the catheter which is not in the bladder is
connected to a lengthy piece of plastic tubing. This in turn is
sealed into a plastic bag that is emptied from time to time.

If the catheter is not left in the bladder, one may be inserted if you are unable to pass sufficient urine after the operation.

The Night Before Your Operation . . .

One of the nurses will measure your legs for some special stockings which will help to improve your circulation for the first few days after the operation.

If you are having an abdominal hysterectomy, the lower part of your abdomen and pubic area will need to be shaved. The hair will grow back to its normal state in due course.

The nurse may give you an enema or suppository to make sure that your bowel is as empty as possible.

You will be offered some form of sedation but the decision whether to take it or not is yours.

No food or drink will be allowed from midnight.

The Day of the Operation

On the morning of your operation you will be asked to go for a bath or shower. Use only soap and water and do not use talcum powder afterwards, as this could clog the clean areas.

Remove all traces of nail varnish, and take out any dentures. You can do this just before going down to theatre if you feel uncomfortable without them.

Do not apply any lipstick.

If you have a wedding ring, it will be covered with a piece of tape. Remove any other jewellery.

Now that you are as clean as possible prior to your operation, a nurse will dress you in a special gown, socks and cap and ask you to stay in bed.

About one hour before, you will be given prescribed pre-medication: this is an injection (usually Valium) after which you will feel drowsy, relaxed and rather dry and thirsty. A name tag will be attached to one of your wrists.

In due course, two hospital porters will wheel you out of the ward, either on your own bed or on a special trolley, and, accompanied by one of the nurses, take you to the ANAESTHETIC ROOM just outside the operating theatre. Final checks are taken to make sure you are the right person on the operating list. The anaesthetist will reassure you as he admin-isters an intravenous injection of anaesthetic, usually into one of the veins on the back of your hand. The injection works very quickly and you will be out like a light before you can count to five . . .

> *. . . unlike Mary Moulden who, in 1828, was given two ounces of gin during her operation and the same amount after its conclusion, with the addition of 60 drops of tincture of opium.*

From there you are wheeled into the OPERATING THEATRE.

Hysterectomy can be undertaken in three ways:

1. **By abdominal incision.** A cut is made horizontally along the top of your pubic hairline: this will leave a slight scar, which will fade in time and become inconspicuous. Sometimes the incision is a vertical one, from below your navel to to the top of your pubic hairline: an incision such as this is necessary if you have large fibroids or an enlarged ovarian cyst. It may be suggested if you have had children born by Caesarean section, so that the incision follows the same scar line on your abdomen.
2. **Vaginally.** The uterus is removed through your vaginal canal, so there is no incision on your abdomen and no scar. A prolapsed uterus is removed this way.
3. **Laparoscopic assisted vaginal hysterectomy (LAVH).** Two small incisions are made in the abdomen, one almost in the navel and the other near the pubic hairline. A laparo-scope is inserted in the incision in the navel, while another instrument is inserted in the second incision. This second instrument loosens the organs to be removed and they are then withdrawn vaginally.

Operations are a team event. There is the consultant surgeon, a first assistant (usually a trainee specialist registrar), nurses, and maybe a senior house officer (SHO) in training. If the oper-ation is being performed in a teaching hospital, the surgeon may either stop halfway through and hand over to the trainee, or share the operating procedures with him/her. There may also be observers present, such as postgraduate student gynaecologists or student doctors. All are intent on applying their medical skills and attention as they help you through this procedure safely.

At the end of the operation, which usually takes about an hour, the hospital porters wheel you into the RECOVERY WARD where you will be closely observed by the nursing staff as you recover from the anaesthetic. You will then return to your own ward once the doctor is satisfied with your progress.

The rest of the day will pass in a haze of sleepiness and waking as you float in and out of consciousness. Your mouth will feel dry, and your throat could be sore where it has been rubbed by the tube going down into your lungs, but you will be given nothing to eat or drink.

This is a busy time for the nursing staff: you will be on half-hourly observation, your blood pressure and pulse will be checked as well as blood loss from your vagina, into which packs will have been inserted to stop any haemorrhage. The nurses will give you regular pain-killing injections, and these will also stop you from feeling sick.

Yet nursing is more than that. A good deal is about creating the right environment, communicating caring warmth from one human being to another. In relation to you, a nurse in many ways fulfils the role of 'mother': she is here at your time of sickness when you have regressed to the level of a needy 'child', a position of extreme vulnerability. The tone of voice, the warmth of her personality, the attention to the detail of your comfort are of great significance as is any informal, physical contact – a hug, holding your hand when the pain is bad, even 'soothing your fevered brow'. With this support through all the following pain, sweat and tears comes the awakening of your will to recover.

The Days after your Operation

The FIRST day is usually the worst. One of the nurses will help you with a wash and the most that you will do is get out of bed and sit in a chair while your bed is remade. When moving or coughing, place both hands over the site of the wound to support it – your stitches will not burst as you move, though coping with attached tubes can seem daunting. Even this small amount of movement is tiring, and you may well sink back into bed exhausted. You may be allowed small sips of water, which will gradually increase until you are drinking normally.

During the day, try and maintain your deep breathing and ankle/foot exercises.

By the SECOND day, you should be feeling more human. You can have a wash in bed or even walk to the bathroom – it depends how you feel. Whether you can walk back is another matter, but you can take this at your own pace, and in most hospitals a wheelchair is available.

If you are able to go to the lavatory, you will need a nurse to take you there, for support – and she will probably advise you not to lock the door, in case you feel dizzy when you stand up again and need to call for help.

There will be pain now that the initial injections of pain relief have worn off. Your skin has been cut, so it will hurt around the site of the wound. But it is not only that which causes pain – the pelvic area internally has been traumatised. Organs such as the bladder and bowel have been disturbed and pushed around during the hysterectomy, and are therefore bruised and tender.

IF YOU NEED PAIN RELIEF, ASK FOR IT. There is no need to be long-suffering. If necessary, make a fuss.

In some hospitals, patients undergoing abdominal surgery are linked to a device containing analgesics, which enables them to self-regulate their pain relief as and when they need it. However, if there is one universal post-hysterectomy experience which causes more distress and tearfulness than any other it is WIND.

The problem of wind got the better of me. I was unprepared – I could have dealt with the expected but not the unexpected. Linda (Croydon)

It is common to suffer wind from the SECOND or THIRD day as gases have built up in your intestines and cannot escape in the normal way, that is, through the bowel, until this is functioning properly. The nurses will dispense a 'peppermint cocktail' and the following remedies are helpful:

- Charcoal tablets
- Mint tea
- Yoghurt
- Mineral water
- Lucozade and soda

You will feel much better once the wind starts to shift, though it will not happen all at once – you have been warned!

Bowels

Because of the bowel preparation before the operation, and the fact that you have had no food to eat for two days, it may be three to four days before your bowels move. A laxative can be prescribed for you to help this; even so it may take time to get sluggish bowels working.

It is not unusual to feel tired and mentally low at this time, and you may suddenly find yourself weeping for no apparent reason. By now, you are unlikely to have either a drip or a drain, so that the very close care and attention has been withdrawn: you may be suffering from delayed shock – or relief that the operation is over and you have come through it safely. Certainly, many women experience unexplained and inexplicable weeping after the birth of a baby, so an hormonal reaction is to be expected when reproductive organs are involved in another major event in a woman's life.

Do not suffer in silence if it helps to talk things through – the doctors and nurses are well aware of this reaction to surgery.

Unless there are any setbacks, you will find yourself improving every day from now on, whether it is resting (either in your own bed or in the day room), enjoying a bath, getting to know others in your ward and taking meals together in the dining room. In all this, you are setting the pace that is right for you.

On pages 114–117 there is a series of simple exercises to improve your muscle tone and strengthen your pelvic area.

Visitors

Nowadays, visiting hours are more flexible in many hospitals, which can make it difficult if you are tired or find it hard to ask family and friends to go. Usually one of the nurses realises this and will tactfully suggest to visitors they come again another day.

A regular visitor, however, will be the consultant or a member of his/her team, to check your daily progress and alleviate any problems. You will be discharged from hospital once this progress is being maintained satisfactorily.

STITCHES or CLIPS hold the wound together and these will be removed when, on inspection, the wound is seen to be healed – any time from five to ten days after the operation. The nurse will do this on the ward, and although you feel her touching you, it should not be painful. Sometimes there is no need for stitches to be removed as the surgeon has placed thread under the skin which will be absorbed.

There may be complications, such as those listed below, which are not resolved before you leave hospital, but you will be given advice about them.

- Difficulty in passing water if no catheter has been used or after the catheter has been taken out. There may be a scalding sensation which indicates a urine infection, so you will be given antibiotics. Sometimes there are repeated urinary infections, and these can be very debilitating.
- Bruising under the skin, also called haematoma (a clot of blood). Occasionally it is necessary to remove a stitch to let a haematoma out.
- Infection in the wound. This can occur if something is not properly sterilised in the operating theatre, or through a drain being used, or if the surgeon takes insufficient care – or purely by chance.

Whatever your experience of this time in your life, you are leaving hospital having undergone a major change which will have a profound effect on the rest of your life. You may be outwardly cheerful, determined to put it all behind you and resume life as before – yet it is during the following few weeks, as you recover your health, that you will need to analyse your thoughts, beliefs and expectations of the operation.

Chapter Five

Progress Towards Recovery

I took the full three months' sick leave which the doctor suggested – I think taking the full time for convalescence is most important. Isobel (Ross-shire)

You need a positive approach to the operation and to realise it does take time for a full recovery. Jackie (Kettering)

Your progress to recovery will happen in stages and is unique for every woman. A successful recovery will be influenced by the following:

- The *skill* of the surgeon and the quality of hospital care.
- Your *physical health* before the operation: it is to your advantage if you are a reasonable weight, have maintained a healthy eating style and do not smoke.
- Your *mental health*: if you are happy about the decision to have the operation, and see it as providing long-term benefits and understand that there will be transitory difficulties.
- Your *domestic back-up*: partners/parents/children who are sensitive, supportive and encouraging will speed up the healing process.
- Your *social back-up*: friends and neighbours who give practical help, leave you to snooze when you are exhausted, and offer a listening ear/shoulder to cry on.

● Your *access* to written information as well as verbal support from a hysterectomy contact (see Useful Addresses, page 148).

Discharge from Hospital

The length of your stay in hospital depends on how quickly you recover. Few patients leave before five days and not many stay in for more than ten days. Healing rates vary with individuals – cuts and grazes take a variable time to heal in different people. At this stage an abdominal scar is purple/bright pink, and as recovery progresses, so this will fade.

On discharge, you may be given one of the following:

● A letter for your GP if you need any follow-up care
● Written information about the 'do's and don'ts' of getting better.

On the other hand, you may leave hospital with nothing other than verbal instructions about your recovery.

First impressions

The anaesthetic and effects of the operation will have a confusing effect when you step outside for the first time. For a few days, relatively speaking, you have been fed, clothed and washed, and decisions have been made for you. Emerging into the real world is an unnerving transition from being a patient to a patient/person.

Convalescence

Years ago, time spent in a convalescence home after surgery was not unusual. Now, whether or not the subject is suggested seems to depend on the view of the consultants, some of whom see it as unnecessary, while others make sure that all their patients are offered the opportunity. The benefits available to all women in Germany were clearly outlined in Sally's experience:

After leaving hospital, I set off for a four-week convalescence period in the Black Forest. This was in a home for 'tired mothers' – any mother with a large family or other tribulations can apply for a 'cure', generally a four–six week stay in such a house. After this good rest, which was accompanied by treatment for my sluggish condition (underwater massage with a stiff brush, alternating hot and cold water and 'water treading') I went home ready to get on with daily life again. We had no extra household help – we could have had a paid home help if any of the children had been under eight years old.

Most women in this country return home, some of them having to cope completely on their own, others using a mixture of methods as they struggle back to normality.

My mum helped for two weeks, then my husband for one week. After that I was on my own but coped because my husband took over at weekends. Mary (Doncaster)

I wish I had money. I would like to have a place where women can recover after the operation. Jean (Essex)

My mother took myself and the children home to her house for a week and I did nothing but rest. Sue (Dorset)

I asked for a home help when I came out of hospital as I was unable to cope with a boisterous two-year-old but could not get any kind of help at all. Eileen (South Yorkshire)

Step-by-Step

Many of the contributors to my questionnaire commented that they would have liked more practical and specific information about convalescence. I agree. We were told 'Take it easy (lie in bed all day?), don't lift anything heavy (an empty kettle? a full one? a bag of potatoes? a baby/toddler/animal?), you'll be back to normal in no time' (really? . . . what does that actually mean?).

It is possible to be specific about certain aspects of recovery, so I have designed a 'step-by-step' plan which shows you and your partner/family how recovery is a very gradual process.

STEP 1 Days 1–4 No domestic chores whatsoever.
Lie down for at least one hour a day.
Listen to your body/mind/spirit – if it wants to go to sleep, then do so, for you will have less energy than you thought.
Try to maintain the gentle mobility exercises outlined on pages 114–117.
Enjoy a daily bath.
Go to bed early.

STEP 2 Days 5–7 Lie down for at least one hour a day.
Help with the washing up and/or dusting but avoid stretching and bending.
Sit down and peel potatoes.
Go for a five-minute walk.
Continue with the exercises.
Go to bed early.

STEP 3 Weeks 2–3 Gradually increase walking. Stop if you feel tired.
Increase the rest periods rather than resting most of the time and being active occasionally.
Light shopping, such as newspaper/magazines/cards can be undertaken.
No bending or lifting of furniture, suitcases, full saucepans, shopping. Do not make the beds.
Try lifting a kettle of water or 1.2-litre/2-pint bottle of squash – stop if there is any pain.
Maintain the exercises.

STEP 4 Weeks 3–4 Start moderate activity – going to the shops and some light shopping, i.e. bread/milk/newspaper.
Help with the washing up and/or dusting.
Go for car rides. (Check that your Insurers are happy about this as some do not approve of driving for 4–6 weeks.) If you feel uncomfortable in the front seat, place a cushion between tummy and seat belt.
Rest if you feel tired.
No bending or lifting, as previous weeks.
Maintain the exercises.

STEP 5 Weeks 4–5 Vacuuming can be attempted if an upright machine is used.
Driving a car is possible, providing you can brake suddenly without abdominal discomfort.
Start routine housework.
Listen to your body/mind/spirit – if you feel tired, then rest with your feet up.
Start bending gently, but not to the floor, and maintain exercises.

STEP 6 Weeks 5–6 Vacuuming can be tried using a cylinder machine.
Add bed-making to the normal household routine.

Exercises for your Abdominal Muscles

These exercises can be attempted from approximately Day 4 onwards. Initially, you may feel too tired to try them more than once or twice but you will feel the benefits if you persist with them. They concentrate on strengthening your stomach muscles so as to avoid future postural and back problems.

Each exercise should be repeated ten times and performed three times daily. Increase the number as your muscles get stronger.

Knee rocking

Lying flat on your back with both knees bent up, let both knees drop first to the left, then to the right within the limits of your pain (five times each side).

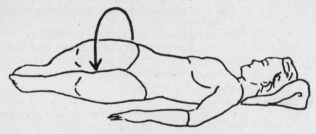

Hip hitching

Lie flat on your back with your head on your pillow, one leg straight and the other one bent. Pull in your tummy and feel your back touching the mattress and HOLD. Now pull your straight leg up at the hip, towards your shoulder, and then stretch down as far as possible. Relax. Change the position of your legs and repeat (five times each side).

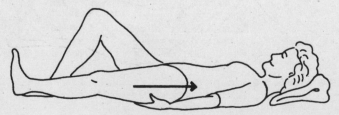

Side bending

Lie flat on your back with your head on your pillow and your legs straight out, then slide your right hand down your right leg – keep your back in contact with your bed. Repeat with your left hand (five times each side).

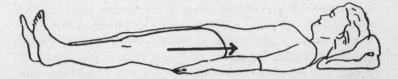

Pelvic tilting

Lie on your bed with one pillow under your head and with both knees bent and together. Press the middle of your back hard down into the mattress by pulling in your tummy muscles and tightening your buttocks as you tilt your bottom upwards. Hold for a slow count of six seconds and release. Repeat five times.

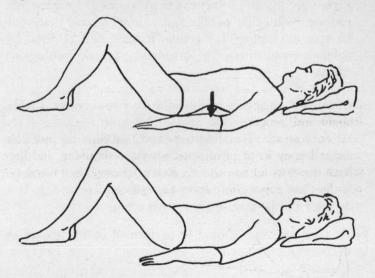

Pelvic Floor Exercises

The pelvic floor is the term used to describe an intricate and strong mesh of muscles which supports the contents of your abdomen.

In women, the pelvic muscles support the vagina. The tube of the vagina is just behind the urethra, so that the muscular support is not strong. These muscles will be affected as a result of an abdominal operation, so pelvic floor exercises concentrate on strengthening the muscles that control closure of the urethra (the opening of the bladder), the vagina and the anus (back passage). If they are weak, this will lead to various degrees of incontinence and prolapse – weakness of these muscles is very common, especially in menopausal women. When they are in good shape, the nerve endings in your vagina will be more easily stimulated, and a sexual climax is more likely to occur.

The following can be practised anywhere, at any time, whether you are sitting, standing or lying down.

1. Remember the time when you used tampons? Imagine that you are with other people and you are aware that your tampon is slipping. Try getting it back into position by tightening and lifting the surrounding muscle inside your vagina.
2. Tighten the muscles from your back passage round to the front, pull up inside you – hold for five seconds – relax slowly and repeat.
3. When you are 'spending a penny', squeeze the muscles around your front passage as tightly as you can, holding back the flow. Count to four slowly, then release the flow. If the flow stops completely, the muscles are strong. If it dribbles a little, then practise more often!

Pelvic floor exercises should be performed by all women at least 20 times daily.

Advanced Abdominal Exercises

These are best performed on the floor.

1. One month after your operation: lie on your back, knees bent up. Lift your head and shoulders off the floor and reach towards your knees (10 x 4 times a day).

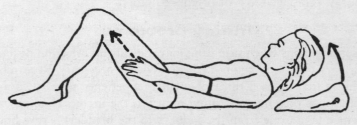

and

2. as (1) above, but stretch diagonally, i.e. left hand to right knee and vice versa (10 x 4 times a day).
3. Two months after your operation: lie on your back, knees bent up. Lift your head, shoulders and back off the floor and reach to your knees (10 x 20 times a day).

and

4. As (3) above, but stretch diagonally, left hand to right knee and vice versa (10 x 20 times a day).

Sporting Activities

Different sports obviously put different stresses on your body. As a general rule, you should wait at least two months before you return to sport, though swimming, which is an excellent way of improving your overall stamina, tone and fitness, can be started six weeks after your operation.

Common Problems

As you rest, take in nourishment and gather strength, physical recovery may encompass some or all of the following problems:

Vaginal discharge

It is quite normal to have a bloodstained or yellowy discharge soon after the operation as the internal stitches dissolve, so you will need to use sanitary pads. The discharge may stop after a couple of weeks, or it may continue for as long as ten weeks. A smelly discharge usually indicates there is an infection, so it should be checked with your GP, as should any heavy, prolonged loss of bright red blood.

Urinary problems

Burning pains when urinating may indicate an infection of the urinary tract, and again medical advice is necessary. Research shows that up to a third of women experience urinary complications post-hysterectomy: injury to the ureters (fine tubes which take urine from the kidneys to the bladder) is rare but can occur, even in the most skilled surgical hands, and slight leaking of urine may initially be present owing to lack of muscle tone. This should settle down in time.

The only complication I had was the constant leak coming from a small tear in one of my ureters . . . it spontaneously repaired itself six weeks after the operation. Anne (Derbyshire)

It's considered normal to have one or even two urinary infections but I feel something happened during surgery because I am now in the fifth week of the fourth course of antibiotics, and have pain constantly in my back. Hilary (Weston-Super-Mare)

I suffered very much with a kidney infection which stubbornly refused to clear up for two to three weeks – unfortunately infections, either external or internal, were all too common in the hospital I attended. Pamela (Cardiff)

Bowel complications

These can be highly distressing, embarrassing and debilitating and at their worst, range from chronic constipation to irritable bowel syndrome. A high fibre diet, with lots of salads, fresh vegetables, raw fruits and brown wholemeal bread, rather than sweet stodgy foods, can encourage sluggish bowels to work again. Drink plenty of fluids – water is still best – particularly when starting to eat more fibre. Water, whether taken from the tap or with added sparkle (i.e. bottled spring water) speeds up kidney activity, and on average, six pints a day should cleanse your system.

I made a dreadful mistake the first night home: my husband bought a Chinese takeaway for all of us – totally the wrong kind of food! Having cured my constipation in hospital, the pains started up again after the Chinese meal. My GP wouldn't come to see me but did suggest Milk of Magnesia, and with my husband dispatched to the chemist, relief was on its way. Monica (Sussex)

I recovered fairly well from the operation itself but suffered badly from irritable bowel syndrome, presumably triggered by the disease (endometriosis), the antibiotics or the operation. This was not diagnosed until eight months later. Jenny (Reading)

Weight gain

Surgery alone will not cause this, but a combination of overeating, lack of exercise and boredom during the recovery phase is a lethal cocktail, especially if you are prone to putting on weight easily. However, I am not convinced that these are the only reasons for weight gain as not enough is known about the effect of major gynaecological surgery on a woman's hormonal system.

I have put on 15 lb (2.7kg) and I'm finding it very difficult to shift, even though I've changed my diet. Ann (Bristol)

Before the operation in March, I could lose weight very easily, but now I've put on a lot and it just won't go, even though I'm being careful. Susan (Newport)

If you are concerned about your increase in weight, prepare a diet diary. Keep it for a week and cover the who, what, when, why and where of your food intake.

Set it up the following way: take a separate page for each day of the week and on each page line up columns with the following headings:

- Time you ate
- What food you consumed
- How much you ate
- What you were doing when you ate
- Where you ate
- With whom you ate, or if alone
- How you felt when you ate.

Keeping this record will make you much more aware of what you really eat and the psychological stimuli associated with your food intake.

You will find yourself very preoccupied with regaining a physical equilibrium, and unable really to consider your feelings about your hysterectomy. And that is quite normal, for to undertake this in a physically weakened state is not possible.

TIREDNESS, EXHAUSTION and TEARS are all part of a normal recovery. But it can seem baffling if this is not quite the scenario painted by the specialist when he pronounced 'You'll be a new woman in six weeks'.

My emotions are extreme at the moment: one day I'm on a high and feel great, the next I'm at rock bottom. These days I try and keep out of everyone's way for fear of bursting into tears. Pauline (West Midlands)

I feel tearful a lot of the time as I was on my own most of the day, and when they came home, my two offspring argued about who was going to do what. But the hardest part was having to keep asking them to do things for me when I could see they wanted to get on with their own lives. Ann (Bristol)

But tears for some women can become more frequent, their feelings of unhappiness compounded by bouts of anxiety and sadness. Painful thoughts can intrude on daily life: for instance, never again having a period . . . never again being able to conceive . . . or maybe saddest of all, never even having one child. You may feel unhappy because you did not have enough information at the time when the decision was made to have the hysterectomy, or that you were somehow deprived of the right to decide for yourself and that perhaps it could have been avoided. Now it is too late.

You may well feel confused, especially if you have completed your family. The relief of no further periods may suddenly seem a heavy price to pay for loss of child-bearing potential, even if you did not really want another child – and you may hesitate to voice these feelings. But it is important that you do so: for you are entering a stage of recovery in which the implications of 'loss' and 'gain' need to be clarified and accepted.

In any hysterectomy there will be feelings of loss, and a time of grieving is needed to acknowledge these and work them through. If you are able to weep angrily/sadly into the sympathetic 'listening ear' of family and friends (even if they do not fully understand your grief), then your sadness and distress will lessen.

It is hard, I think, to explain the sense of loss I felt in the early post-op stages. I had a loving partner and three fine teenage sons, yet something very important to me had been taken away. Christine (London)

I recovered well after excellent care in hospital, and I was determined to be positive, to get on with my life. Which was fine until two months later when I suddenly went to pieces. I went to stay with a friend and poured it all out – I know now that this should have happened earlier. Sue (Brighton)

Although I had to have the operation, the guilt of my daughter being an only child and the sorrow of no more babies is often too dreadful to bear. Stephanie (West Yorkshire)

Self-help

Several of my correspondents wrote long letters detailing their medical/life histories before and after hysterectomy, adding that they had found it therapeutic to write it all down.

Buy a large lined notepad, and if you are not sure where to begin, consider the following outline:

- When your menstrual problems started
- The treatment you were given, its effectiveness or otherwise
- The impact on yourself, and how it affected your personal life
- The decision to have a hysterectomy and your hospital experience
- Your thoughts and feelings now – what you have lost and what you have gained.

If your hysterectomy has been for cancer, you are childless and had wanted a baby, your writing could take the form of a 'Letter to my unborn child' telling your 'child' about yourself, your family, your hopes and dreams, and what you might have shared and enjoyed together.

You may decide to write this all at once, or gradually over a few weeks. Once it is finished, put all the pages in a large envelope and tuck them away at the back of a drawer. Alternatively, you may find it easier to express yourself in drawing and painting. You will need two sheets of white paper, and again if you are not sure where to begin, the following should help:

- Draw/paint an image of yourself before the hysterectomy: you might be curled up in pain on a bed, or huddled miserably in a chair. Around you, draw/paint things which you needed when it was really bad, such as hot water bottles, extra towels, Disprin/pain-killers/anti-depressants, etc.
- If you have a partner, add a picture of him/her in relation to you at this time. You might want to draw/paint several

images – one showing sympathy (an arm around your shoulder), another anger (shouting at you) or exhaustion (head in hands).

● If you have a child or children, add them to the picture, and if relevant, include people you know at work.

You may find yourself using a lot of black and red paint to indicate the feelings and emotions around at the time.

By now, you will have a composite picture of yourself before the operation. Put it out of sight before you begin the next picture on the second piece of paper, and this will show how you see yourself and your life now.

Once it is complete, compare the two pictures – are they very different? – and put them away somewhere safe in an envelope.

When physical recovery and a grieving and working through of emotions have taken place, there remains a final stage of adjustment which might be termed conceptual, intellectual, or even philosophical in nature. This is when the hysterectomy is reviewed once more, on a more objective mental level. Questions are raised such as 'Why me? Why should I have gone through this trauma?' Answers are found such as 'Why NOT me? Why should I be immune from problems?' A mental acceptance is made of the new state of your body – a verbal statement confirms it: 'This is me. What am I going to do now?'

A new concept of self-image must be formed which incorporates your body loss in proper perspective. If you are feeling very badly about your new image, you may use words like 'mutilated' when speaking of yourself. You may describe yourself as 'empty', 'having a vast hole within'. It is true that organs have been removed, but it is possible to see your body after surgery as healthy and normal in every function, except one – you cannot conceive and carry a child. You will still be all the things you were before, once the loss of child-bearing is accepted.

If you are feeling *good* about your new image, you may

describe yourself as 'relieved', 'free', and 'in control'. Confronting yourself in a full-length mirror shows the same body (even if the tummy muscles are a little loose), a body no longer governed by menstrual bleeding, pain, mood swings, tiredness and ill-health.

So when self-image is correctly perceived, the concept of self-esteem – the value you place on yourself – can be adjusted to accept the fact of hysterectomy. Now you may well feel a new pride and strength in your ability to cope with, and emerge from, an assault on your physical and emotional health.

If you have used the SELF-HELP ideas, this is the time to take out the envelope of writings and/or paintings, and dispose of them – after all, you don't need them now, do you?

My operation was the best thing that could have happened, even though I was terrified beforehand. It opened up a new life for me, as I was so ill before. Janet (Suffolk)

It's great being able to do things when I want without checking the calendar first. Gillian (Kent)

It sounds odd but one of the things I've enjoyed most is buying and keeping good underwear. I was always ruining mine in spite of wearing pads. Janet (London)

Sex after Hysterectomy

Many women are concerned about their sexual response after removal of their uteri – will their sex drive change? will they experience orgasms? and will their partners notice anything different?

They are right to be concerned. Even if they do not fully understand what their sexual organ looks like inside, they suspect that taking part of it away must make a difference to sexual pleasure.

That there are no clear-cut answers to these concerns is shown when considering the following circumstances.

Where are you coming from?

Sexual desire is an appetite or drive present in all of us in varying degrees. But our understanding of ourselves as sexual beings is shaped in part by exposure to the following influences:

1. **Parental.** Adults in your home hugged and kissed each other naturally, there were compliments and comfortings between them. There was affection shown to you (and any siblings) as well as help and praise. Anxieties, hurts and disappointments were shared as much as jokes and laughter, and angry arguments were sorted out openly. Valued and respected, you emerged with a fair degree of confidence into your adult life.

   Conversely, your home may have been outwardly respectable and inwardly cheerless: watchful of adult tensions, you became confused and uncertain as occasional affection was interspersed with cold withdrawal. Your natural curiosity was answered by embarrassment or hostility, and by your teens you were self-contained and suspicious, unable to trust anyone.

2. **Social.** A social life, whether at school, in work or at play, offers different perspectives of sexual behaviour ranging from flirtation, teasing and petting to sexual aggression and unwelcome advances. Some of this may have alarmed you, yet you gradually gained confidence in sexual expression. On the other hand, maybe you felt shy and uncertain socially, frightened of being rejected, so that you were unable to risk any intimacy, even as you longed for a close relationship.

3. **Cultural.** Perhaps women's role within your culture was dependent on fertility, and the ability to conceive and bear a child seen as a measure of 'womanhood'. This might be especially frightening for you if you are unable to live up to these expectations, or your partner believes you will be less of a woman after hysterectomy. Within a wider cultural perspective, the portrayal of women in society could have reinforced or demoralised your self-esteem.

4. **Religious.** For many faiths, deviation from prescribed sexual conduct is regarded as a sin: virginity may be seen as a prerequisite of marriage, chemical contraception and abortion forbidden, while for some, adultery is punishable by stoning. The conflict between beliefs and reality may have resulted in painful decisions for you.

You may have recognised yourself in some of this, perhaps even been surprised to realise how much these influences have affected your sexual experiences.

Where are you now?

A further influence on your sexual development has been your menstrual cycle. Hundreds of my respondents wrote about this, in sorrow and in anger: a catalogue of symptoms – PMT, flooding (which wrecked clothes and bedding), tiredness, migraines, chronic pain, sudden and heavy bleeding, sleeping on bath towels, using sanitary pads and tampons. All of these contributed to sexual frustrations, broken relationships and disruption of work, studies and holidays. Maybe this is 'where you are now'.

Or you may have enjoyed a sexually active partnership, assuming a longed-for pregnancy, but have started bleeding between your periods – a smear test has revealed cell abnormalities.

Perhaps sex had been satisfying until recently when your periods became heavier and there was uncomfortable pressure on your bladder: diagnosis shows that there are two fibroids in your uterus. These have been monitored over the months and are growing rapidly, hence the recommendation of hysterectomy.

It is this subtle blending of emotional and physical contact which determines your sexual pleasure, for good sex is certainly not a matter of mechanics. In addition, sexual relationships are constantly being readjusted to take account of the degree of risk of pregnancy, the method of contraception (if used), and stressful life events such as birth, feared or real unemployment, disablement and bereavement.

Where might you be post-operatively?

Most women feel tired and indifferent to sex after hysterectomy and it is not unusual for interest to return gradually.

What you will need is to have your confidence restored as a woman, to know you are loved with or without a womb. If you have a loving partner, from the first night of getting home from hospital, get close to each other: tender loving care, gentle stroking, thoughtful concern and comforting are needed during this healing process.

If sexual intercourse is part of your lives together, then it is wise not to attempt it until at least six weeks after the operation: penetration soon after surgery can cause bleeding from the internal suture line at the top of your vagina and you could run the risk of infection.

Sexual arousal

You know what triggers your special response – whispered endearments . . . the light fingertip tracery on smooth skin . . . the smell of your partner . . . a glass of sparkling wine . . . tenderness . . . Both of you may well feel apprehensive the first time, so try and talk about your fears and anxieties. Take your time. If your vagina appears to need moistening, either you or your partner can gently apply some K-Y jelly with a finger.

As your bodies respond to each other, extra blood begins to flow causing your genitals to swell. Your vagina will become moist with a natural lubricant produced by the blood vessels in its tissues. Your vagina swells, so that instead of it being its usual length (8–10cm/3½–4 inches), it is temporarily increased to 13 or 15cm/5 or 6 inches, and it is the outer part of your vagina (the first third) which is highly sensitive to touch of any kind.

Sexual Enjoyment and orgasm

Women differ. You may be breast sensitive, or vaginally sensitive, or you may be provoked to orgasm by stimulation of your clitoris. Or you may be a woman who needs deep vaginal penetration to secure a type of satisfaction which differs from that provided by stimulation of your vagina and clitoris.

On a physiological level, every orgasm is the same: the tension and congestion in the pelvis caused by the stimulation of a vast network of nerves is released in orgasm. But it can feel different. Sensations will vary in intensity depending on the changing level of excitement and the level of arousal, as well as general health and hormone balance.

The loss of your uterus and cervix may not make any difference to your orgasm if you experience vaginal contractions at the moment of release. But the uterus and cervix are part of your female sex organ. The uterus elevates during the excitement phase of intercourse and contracts during orgasm, and while many women are unaware of this, some are aware.

In an informative article in 1981 in the American Journal of Obstetrics and Gynecology, the late Dr Leon Zussman summed up the pertinent research about post-hysterectomy responsiveness and the uterus:

> *For some women, the quality of orgasm is related to the movement of the uterus and the cervix, and for these women the intensity of orgasm is thus diminished when these structures are removed. For other women, orgasm is achieved mainly by clitoral stimulation so that the loss of the internal structures does not have a comparable effect. Evidence that women experience one or both types of orgasm, sometimes blended, has been reported over many years and conforms with our clinical observations. The percentage of women for whom the cervix and uterus are important is unknown.*

Dr Zussman added that it was difficult to predict the sexual outcome after hysterectomy. Research has shown that an equal number of women experienced increased sexual desire as experienced a diminution in sex drive, and this is borne out by these extracts from my questionnaires.

> *I had my hysterectomy seven years ago and have been numb since then. I have no sexual feelings at all, though I still have my ovaries. I cannot find out why I am left like this.* Susan (Belfast)

It took me all of six months to start feeling anything like normal. Except for my love life. That started back in a minor way (masturbating) just one week after the operation. I think my boyfriend was trying to tell me that I was just the same. It was very good but I was told later that orgasmic contractions might not do me any good, and that I should avoid them. (I think catching up on the neglected housework did me more harm). Ann (Bristol)

My worst problem before hysterectomy was pre-menstrual tension, which was almost non-stop. The physical side was terrible and I could hardly allow my husband to touch me, therefore our sex life suffered almost irreparably. After the operation – I can't explain why – my PMT totally disappeared. My husband and I now enjoy a wonderful sex life which has probably saved our marriage. Pauline (West Midlands)

On the first occasion of sexual intercourse, I chickened out right at the last moment, but my husband was gentle and understanding – I think he was as scared as I was. The next time it worked beautifully, the only problem I had was psychological. It's difficult to explain, but I felt it was rather like tonic without the vodka – as though he wasn't going into me, the fundamental me, just a tube left by the surgeon. Luckily I was able to talk to my husband about this, and he reassured me that it felt just the same as ever, even better because he knew he wasn't going to hurt me, whereas in the past he'd been worried that he might be causing me pain or further damage. This feeling soon passed, and by the time I returned to hospital for my check-up, our sex life was as good as it had always been. Ann (Clwyd)

One thing bothers me now and that is where the incision was made four years ago – across the bikini line – there is no feeling whatsoever, and hasn't been since the operation. Mavis (Halifax)

Recovering natural sexual responsiveness can take up to a year after hysterectomy. There is evidence that over 40 per cent of women report decreased sexual response after hysterectomy-oophorectomy. For years, it has been believed that this is psychogenic, i.e. all in the mind.

> *My doctor told me before the operation that it would make no difference to sex, but it has. I do not have an orgasm or reach a climax and cannot satisfy myself which causes me distress. When I consulted a sex counsellor, she was surprised and said she thought the problem was all in my mind.* Jean (West Midlands)

It is not. It sounds as though stimulation of her cervix, uterus and broad ligaments played an important part in orgasm for Jean so their removal has resulted in a real loss of sexual pleasure. Furthermore, her sexual function may have been affected by damage to the nerves in that region during the operation.

The relatively limited data available thus far suggests, but does not confirm, the possibility that sexual response following genital surgery may be at least partially determined by the constantly circulating, transforming and interdependent hormones. As far back as 1948, research had established that the hormone testosterone enhances libido in women, and today testosterone pellets can provide relief for loss of libido after the menopause.

It is therefore difficult to predict the sexual outcome after hysterectomy, as so many factors contribute to sexual satisfaction.

Chronic Difficulties

For the majority of women who have a hysterectomy the results are successful, and their health is greatly improved. For a few women the reverse is true, and they find themselves facing a new set of problems. This can be especially difficult for them if they know other women who have had a hysterectomy since their own, and who appear to be fully recovered and in good health.

The following conditions require medical help:

Depression

Post-hysterectomy women differ from other post-surgery control groups in being prescribed more anti-depressant drugs, and having more headaches and sleeplessness as well as experiencing more untreated depression. There is a 33 per cent incidence of depression after hysterectomy, compared with a 7 per cent incidence after other abdominal surgery, yet all too often it is suggested that 'it's all in your head', thereby inferring that depressed post-hysterectomy women lack courage or backbone – or both.

Ironically, part of the answer is that it is all in your head, for the metabolism of hormones within the brain is now believed to depend on oestrogen levels. So depression, anxiety and headaches can be alleviated for some women by HRT. But not others, which demonstrates that teasing out the reasons for a condition which can occur at any time up to three years after hysterectomy is complicated.

Depression is more likely to occur under the following circumstances:

- If surgery is necessary and you have not had a child and had hoped to do so
- If response to previous experiences of stress had been a difficulty in coping
- If you are on your own and isolated, with no family and few friends, and have no meaningful focus to your life
- If you are married/in a relationship, and it is not handled with sensitivity
- If you have allowed yourself to become swept up in the decision-making process without either understanding or querying the reasons for the operation.

Nothing went wrong in hospital but I was led to believe I would feel great after six weeks, whereas I still felt terrible. This led to my getting very depressed. Mary (Hemel Hempstead)

Although I accepted the need for the hysterectomy, I did suffer depression for nearly a year afterwards. Kathleen (Middlesex)

All was well until about three months after the operation when I developed severe depression. I have anti-depressants which help when I am really bad, but when the course finishes, I become depressed again with great anxiety and phobias. My GP has given me HRT for hot flushes and dizziness but these were never really a problem. It is now five years on and I have gone from being physically fit with a family, part-time job and many hobbies to feeling I'm an overweight neurotic mess with no great hope of recovery. Jean (Belfast)

There is an agreement that low self-esteem is often associated with various negative psychological experiences including guilt, dissatisfaction with life, depression and withdrawal from social roles. Thus Mary might have felt 'guilty' because she was not conforming to the gynaecologist's prediction of improved health after six weeks, therefore she was 'odd' compared to other women who she assumed were not 'feeling terrible'. It is then but a short step to depression. Whereas Kathleen's depression centred more on her inability to bear children, Jean's aftermath of hysterectomy appears to indicate a hormonal system that has gone completely haywire.

Being depressed is a profoundly emotional experience and its intensity can frighten both sufferer and partner/family/friends. It is often difficult to separate what is physical from what is emotional, and medical help is essential, though this does not necessarily mean a prescription for anti-depressants.

Irritable Bowel Syndrome

Symptoms may include abdominal pain and spasm, diarrhoea, constipation or both, a sharp pain felt low down inside the rectum and involuntary soiling of underwear. Various treatments, including heat treatment, dietary control with bran or isogel, or muscle relaxants can be helpful, as can contacting the IBS Network (see Useful Addresses, page 148).

Urinary symptoms

This may be stress incontinence when coughing, laughing or sneezing, or a continuous leaking of urine. Medication and physiotherapy can be helpful.

Severe back pain

This includes an inability to stand or walk for any length of time. You will need to be patient while trying various forms of treatment, and that is not easy when there seems to be no end to the pain.

Some conditions such as adhesions, pelvic inflammation and endometriosis may recur, and these should be discussed with your GP.

Making a Complaint

There are a number of options available in order to obtain the information you require or to complain about what has happened.

The first is an informal hospital complaint. Speak to the staff nurse, sister or consultant about what has happened, as it is always a good idea to discuss the matter diplomatically. You might want this discussion to be in private and for a friend or relative to be present. If you have been discharged from hospital, you can arrange to talk to your consultant, again in private and with a friend or relative present.

If you obtain no satisfaction from these discussions or from talking to the appropriate hospital administrator, you can then make a formal complaint, and the informal complaint will form the basis of a hospital complaints procedure.

Other options include: complaining to the Health Service Ombudsman, informally approaching the Family Health Services Authority; writing directly to the General Medical Council; or contacting Action for Victims of Medical Accidents (AVMA). (See Useful Addresses, page 148.)

These procedures can seem very daunting when you are recovering post-operatively, so if you are concerned, it would be wise to keep a record of what is happening to you.

I got a sharp pain in my left groin eight days after my operation and after investigation was told there were massive adhesions, that there was nothing that could be done and I would have to live with the pain. Two years on and I am still in a lot of pain – I can't walk more than 50 yards or stand long enough to cook a meal without being in agony . . . I have gone from being very fit – I used to play county netball and run my own playgroup – to being a semi-invalid. The thing that makes me most angry is that the medical authorities just don't want to know. Christine (Kelvedon)

I haemorrhaged five times after the birth of my baby by Caesarean section, so a hysterectomy was performed. Afterwards, we wanted to sue the local hospital but were put in rather an awkward situation: we hoped to adopt another baby, but were given the impression that we could only do one or the other, and as we wanted a child more than compensation, we chose to adopt. Really, all we wanted to know was the truth of what had happened to me which no one was prepared to tell me. Heather (Essex)

Counting the Costs

All surgical procedures carry risk. More than 800 medical accidents happen in NHS hospitals every day, some of which concern gynaecological surgery. That a few of these result in legal action is hardly surprising, for medicine is now accountable for its actions – far more so than when this book was first published in 1993.

The exact percentage of medical accidents is not known at present, but it is unlikely to be more than 2 per cent of all operations, and not all medical accidents involve medical negligence. The simplest way of defining negligence is that it is an accident for which somebody is to blame.

While transitory complications may be acceptable, the long-term effects of errors are another matter. Women have obtained compensation for the removal of a uterus and/or ovaries without consent, while at least one woman received a substantial out-of-court settlement for ongoing incontinence – she underwent 84 operations to try and correct complications after a hysterectomy.

Taking legal action

If you remain dissatisfied with the explanations given, and your condition is not improving, the next stage is to explore the possibility of legal action, but before embarking on this you should consider the following:

- Can you afford the legal costs? If not, and you possess an insurance policy, it is worth checking if there is a clause covering legal costs. Another possibility could be Legal Aid.
- Look in Yellow Pages for solicitors specialising in medical negligence. You could also contact CAB (Citizens Advice Bureau) for a recommendation. Some solicitors offer an initial free half-hour session. Taking this up would give you the opportunity to explore the whole issue.
- Ask the solicitor about his/her experience in handling medical litigation: you need to have some idea as to how successful litigation might or might not be in your circumstances, and how long it might take to resolve the matter.
- Before the appointment, write down all the facts about the situation in as methodical a way as you can and send a copy of it to the solicitor – that way he/she will have some understanding of the situation before you meet.
- Obtain a statement of costs and method of payment. (The likelihood is that the costs could be higher than those stated.)
- Medical litigation is a long drawn-out process which can last several years. Only make a commitment to embark on it once you have assembled all the facts, weighed them up and understand that resolution of your claim is likely to be a long time ahead.

AT PRESENT, THERE IS NO COMPLAINTS PROCEDURE FOR PRIVATE PATIENTS. This applies to private hospitals, private surgeons, physicians, alternative or complementary therapists and private family practitioners. The only available route open is to take legal action by instituting a civil claim for medical negligence. This is extremely expensive and sets the patient against the much greater resources of the medical profession.

A pressure group for change (APROP – see Useful Addresses, page 148) was formed in 1998 and its members are campaigning for tougher legislation within the private healthcare industry.

Chapter Six

The Way Forward

Perhaps you are reading this book because your GP has intimated that a hysterectomy is a possibility, and you want to find out what this means. You may have undergone other gynaecological operations and dislike the idea of another one. Or you believe strongly that any surgical intervention should only be undertaken if your life is in danger – or you feel your uterus is an important part of you, of your individual self, and that its removal will constitute a violation of this self.

Reading the preceding chapters has, I hope, given you information about hysterectomy and the alternatives to it. What might be your next step?

First you need to recognise that your body belongs to no one else but you – and it's the only one you've got! Whatever the advice offered, only you should decide on the form of treatment, for you will be living with the results of that treatment after it is completed.

Having said that, there are some exceptions. The first of these is cancer of the reproductive organs. Invasive cervical cancer is a terrible disease that should be treated immediately by hysterectomy – this can save your life. While there is no direct correlation between cervical cancer and ovarian cancer, if the original cancer has reached the ovaries, then everything must come out. Endometrial cancer is also life-threatening and hysterectomy is the best treatment available. It may have surprised you to read that only 5–10 per cent of hysterectomies in the UK are for cancer of the reproductive organs, but the impact of the cancer is as traumatic as for any form of cancer. This is especially so when it means the loss of potential motherhood.

The second exception concerns women who have a specific physical disability, such as multiple sclerosis, where an alternative treatment such as endometrial ablation might be strongly recommended by the consultant as the recovery time following hysterectomy is very much longer. Of course, if there is a diagnosis of cancer, hysterectomy will have to be performed.

If you are not among these exceptions, then you have a part to play in deciding the best course of action for you. This means carefully considering the following:

- *Where you are personally at this point in time*: with a partner, single, engaged, widowed, divorced/divorcing.
- *Whether your personal life includes children or not*: if it does, have you completed your family? Are the children young? Are they grown up? If you do not have children at present, do you hope for children? Do you *not* want any?
- *Your role(s) in life at present*: working full-time as a homemaker with a family and part-time outside earner . . . working full-time in a responsible, stressful environment (such as teaching) and as a partnered home-maker . . . working full-time as a home-maker with a family that includes an elderly parent and/or child with a disability . . . a divorced parent on Income Support/part-time outside earner . . . working full-time as a divorcing parent and single person home-maker . . . working full-time as a home-maker without children . . . working as a full-time student without children.
- *How your menstrual disorders affect the quality of your life*. You might feel that certain aspects are worse than others, i.e. you can sometimes control the pain but not always . . . you are worried sick when seen in public as you always need to be sure there is a toilet nearby, just in case . . . you have days off work, huddled up with a hot-water bottle . . . sporting activities cannot be enjoyed . . . you are totally fed-up with the monthly 'battle'.

Clarifying all of this is a way of creating a 'personal profile' which only you can do. It might help to write it down.

The next step is to consider the advantages or otherwise of either major surgery (hysterectomy, page 14), minimally invasive surgery (endometrial ablation, pages 38 and 43 / uterine embolisation of fibroids, page 44) or complementary therapy (acupuncture, page 54 / herbalism, page 62 / home-opathy, page 67). You will need to find out whether there are any complementary therapists in your area – and there are medical doctors who also practise acupuncture and homoeopathy (refer to Useful Addresses, page 148).

If you decide to undergo minor surgery discuss it with your GP and ask to be referred to an appropriate consultant.

That leaves hysterectomy, and once you are reasonably sure that this is the right course of action for you, you will become part of a three-person process of some complexity.

Patient/Doctor Communication

You have chosen to take some responsibility for your own health care, and self-responsibility is very important as it should promote an effective partnership between you and the doctors.

Having identified a need for change, this decision will have been influenced by the variety of factors in the early part of this chapter. Discussing it further with your GP will give you the opportunity to explain why you believe hysterectomy is the answer for your menstrual disorders, and to discuss any anxieties outside the remit of my book. For instance, you may have an elderly parent staying with you, so you will need to know whether any domestic help is available while you are recuperating. Not only that, but reading a book or informa-tion leaflet is very different from discussing it face-to-face, especially if there are aspects you still find troubling.

GPs are known to differ widely in their referral thresholds and in their relationships with consultants, and a GP who favours surgery may choose to refer to a consultant who is known to favour surgery – and some GPs may use referral as a way of getting rid of troublesome patients. Lastly, consultants vary in their opinion as to when surgery is indicated.

There is no doubt the consultant represents 'The Authority' to many of us, and we can find ourselves intimidated by this – it takes an assured and articulate woman to voice anxieties during a consultation. Some consultants exhibit an authority because of particular circumstances: I can still recall the uncomfortable feelings evoked in me when talking to my consultant in a tiny examination room which contained one chair in a corner and a couch – I sat on the chair, and he stood leaning against the couch.

Others have seen it all before and regard hysterectomy as such an obvious solution as to merit little explanation. You may feel embarrassed about discussing the more personal and sexual implications of the operation – often the very areas which cause most anxiety – or feel guilty at taking up what you perceive as the consultant's valuable time. It is very easy to think this, but your peace of mind is very important.

Reaction to a recommendation of hysterectomy can range from relief to surprise to shock. You may be relieved that an end is in sight to your menstrual disorders, but it is very different for others who are surprised or shocked – indeed, the consultant may be totally unaware of what they are feeling because these women are stunned into silence. This is compounded because we are all unable to retain or absorb information when we are anxious. That is why taking a friend with you to the consultation could be helpful: both of you will retain something of what has been said, as you are unlikely to be given any written information to take away with you.

Unfortunately, many women find their consultations bewildering. Failure to communicate appropriately may also be a way of a professional retaining power – the expert knows what he or she is doing and assumes the patient has little to offer to the occasion.

My consultant said I should have a hysterectomy for prolapse of my womb, and within minutes I was booked into a clinic for the following Tuesday week. I don't remember walking out and getting home. I was so shocked, I didn't eat for the rest of the day. Anyway, I saw a programme about hysterectomy on TV, rang the number and talked about it all, and I was sent a leaflet. I decided I was not prepared to have a hysterectomy at my age – I am 75 and my husband is 82 – so I am going to have a ring fitted, even though it will have to be changed every few months. Alice (Minehead)

Alice's understanding of the consultation may be totally different from that of the consultant, who might have believed that a direct and firm approach prescribing the appropriate treatment would be accepted as the right one. It doesn't sound as though Alice was even once asked 'How do you feel about this?' which at least would have given her the chance to express some reaction.

Of course, no two consultants act the same way towards their potential hysterectomy patients, but a poor level of communication between consultant and patient is all too common, and is the reason why hysterectomy contacts receive thousands of telephone calls and letters every year asking for information.

A few hospitals offer a hysterectomy counselling service to patients, their partners and families, from the time there is any suggestion that a hysterectomy may be necessary. Until her retirement, Sally Haslett, a nurse at St Thomas' Hospital, London, covered all aspects of advice – counselling before and after surgery and giving specific information with regard to general health and sexual activity following discharge. For many women, simply to discuss sexuality on a professional level is a revelation.

Judging by comments from many of my respondents, there is a need for this counselling service elsewhere.

As an RMN who has worked with patients suffering from clinical depression after hysterectomy, I would advise pre- and post-op counselling. Yvonne (Birmingham)

> *The lack of counselling available and a seeming igno-*
> *rance of psychological implications appalled me and still*
> *does.* Dale (Isle of Wight)

> *I think some kind of post-op counselling would have*
> *been helpful.* Marea (Isle of Man)

> *I felt I desperately needed counselling before and*
> *especially after the operation . . . I received none until I*
> *demanded to be referred, even though I was desperate*
> *and upset. Very few women seem to need long-term*
> *support. One or two sessions seem to be all that is*
> *required – only a few need more, i.e. those who are*
> *young, have cancer or wanted children.* Katie (North
> Berwick)

This hysterectomy counselling service at St Thomas' Hospital
could serve as a role model throughout the UK. It would bring
the following benefits:

- It can take time for the recommendation of hysterectomy
  to be absorbed, so the consultation is not really the right
  time to talk about all the implications.
- A counselling service creates a 'bridge' between consultation and prospective operation.
- An on-going supportive relationship between patient and
  counsellor allows for exploration of issues of concern, as
  well as practical advice and specific information giving.

Finally, one of the aspects which truly appals me is the lack of
after-care: women are discharged after a major operation
without the assurance of at least one home visit. Hysterectomy
is seen as such a commonplace operation, even though every
surgical intervention carries risk. This is in sharp contrast to
childbirth, and while I would not dispute that it is right for a
mother to expect the greatest possible care and attention, hundreds of women are at their most vulnerable during the first
few weeks after hysterectomy. Furthermore, even the six-week
check-up with the consultant is increasingly unusual. Women
are now told to contact their GP if they are worried.

I think a district nurse could call at least once a week to see if you are all right – many women like myself were on their own all day. Mary (Hemel Hempstead)

No one from the medical profession, i.e. GP or a district nurse, came to see me – a couple of visits from a nurse or health visitor would have been beneficial. Linda (Croydon)

My husband is a nurse tutor – however, he wasn't aware of the side-effects. I feel there should be back-up for patients after the operation. Teena (Taunton)

Research shows that thousands of women are delighted with the long-term benefits of hysterectomy, even when some post-operative problems recur or persist for a long time. So many of them write to me about achievements professionally, fulfilling ambitions and finding new directions in their lives, as well as enjoying themselves for the first time in years. It was as if menstruation had shackled them – and now they were free!

I had several remarks such as, 'you're never a real woman after that operation', etc. I think that's a load of rubbish. I have felt fit and well with a great sense of freedom since my hysterectomy. Jeanne (Oxford)

It's changed my life. I have so much more energy and enthusiasm, it increased my confidence and enabled me to plan ahead without the dreaded 'curse'. Judith (Milton Keynes)

Eighteen months after the operation, the scar is barely visible and I feel absolutely marvellous. Vivienne (West Sussex)

The last words belong to Ann of Clwyd. She was my very first correspondent and wrote to me exactly a year after her hysterectomy – her letter encouraged, amused and inspired me.

The main bonus has been the closeness between my husband and me. Having him at home when I came out of hospital made my recovery a joint effort, and when we look back on it now, we remember it as a happy time when we faced difficulty together – and triumphed.

May yours be a triumph as well.

Glossary of Medical Terms

Adenomyosis: A condition in which cells like those in the endometrium are found embedded in the muscular wall of the uterus. It is sometimes called 'internal endometriosis' and is frequently only diagnosed after hysterectomy.

Adhesion: A thick band of scar tissue which can form after any surgery. Patches of scar tissue can extend from one organ to another so that they get stuck together, causing pain and discomfort and preventing the organs from functioning properly.

Anaemia: A pathological deficiency in the haemoglobin (oxygen) in the blood, or in the number of red blood cells.

Bilateral oophorectomy: The surgical removal of both ovaries.

Bilateral salpingo-oophorectomy: The surgical removal of both ovaries and both Fallopian tubes.

Cancer: Malignant growth of cells.

Catheter: A plastic tube inserted into the bladder in order to drain it.

Cervix: The lower part, or neck, of the uterus where it joins the vagina.

Chemotherapy: Drug treatment of cancer.

CIN: The term used in grading pre-cancerous changes of the cervix.

Corpus luteum: A yellow mass formed in the ovary after the egg (ovum) has been released.

Cryocautery: The freezing technique used to destroy the endometrium.

Cyst: A swelling filled with fluid.

Cytotoxic: Destructive to cells.

Dilation and curettage: Usually called a D & C. This is a diagnostic procedure in which samples of the endometrium are removed for examination under a microscope. Often known as a 'scrape'.

Endometrial ablation: The surgical removal of the endometrium using a resectoscope with/without a rollerball electrode, laser, thermal balloon therapy and microwave.

Endometriosis: A disease in which cells present in the endometrium develop in other parts of the pelvis.

Endometrium: The lining of the uterus which grows every month and is shed during menstruation if pregnancy has not occurred.

Epidural: An anaesthetic which is injected into the outer lining of the spinal cord.

Fallopian tubes: The two tubes leading from the uterus to the ovaries.

Fibroids: Lumps of fibrous and muscular tissue, varying in size, which are found on all levels of the uterus.

Haematoma: A clot of blood which can form in an abdominal incision and may become infected.

Haemorrhage: Abnormally high levels of bleeding.

Hormone: A chemical substance produced in minute quantities in one part of the body and circulated to organs by the bloodstream.

Hormone replacement therapy (HRT): A course of hormones in tablet, patch, implant or gel form, prescribed to replace hormones no longer produced naturally by the ovaries.

Hysterectomy: The surgical removal of the uterus.

Hysteroscope: A surgical instrument with a light and telescopic lens at one end.

Laparoscopy: A minor operation using a surgical instrument like a telescope (laparoscope) to examine the organs in the pelvis.

Laparotomy: A major operation which involves opening the abdomen just below the bikini line so that the problems can be assessed.

Ligament: A tough band of fibrous tissue connecting bones or supporting organs within the abdomen.

Menopause: The time in a woman's life when her menstrual cycle ceases.

Menorrhagia: Heavy prolonged bleeding.

Menstrual cycle: The number of days from one menstruation to the next, during which regular hormonal changes occur.

Menstruation: The cyclic discharge of blood from the non-pregnant uterus. Usually it occurs at approximately four-week intervals.

Myomectomy: The surgical removal of fibroids.

Oestrogen: One of the female hormones produced in the ovaries.

Oophorectomy: The surgical removal of one ovary.

Ovaries: The two organs attached to the Fallopian tubes either side of the uterus which produce eggs (ova) and hormones.

Ovulation: The time during each month when one or two eggs (ova) are released from the ovaries.

Progesterone: A female hormone produced by the corpus luteum. It thickens the lining of the uterus in preparation for a fertilised egg.

Progestogen: A synthetic form of the hormone progesterone.

Prolapse: The displacement of any organ from its normal position.

Radiotherapy: The treatment of cancer using high-energy rays.

Resectoscope: A thin viewing surgical instrument with a small wire loop at the end of it which is electrically heated.

Salpingo-oophorectomy: The removal of one Fallopian tube and ovary.

Testosterone: A hormone produced by the ovaries.

Tumour: A lump of cells. Tumours can be either benign or malignant. Benign cells do not spread to other parts of the body and so are not cancerous, whereas malignant cancer cells have the ability to spread beyond the original site and, if left untreated, may invade and destroy surrounding tissue.

Ultrasound: A painless diagnostic technique in which the pelvic organs are viewed on a video monitor.

Ureter: The tube carrying urine from the kidney to the bladder.

Uterine artery embolisation: A surgical procedure which cuts off the blood supply to fibroids.

Uterus: Womb.

Vagina: The passage leading from outside the woman's body to the uterus.

Vault: The upper part of the vagina into which the cervix protrudes.

Wertheim's hysterectomy: A more extensive and radical hysterectomy performed for some cases of cancer of the reproductive organs.

Useful Contacts

Enclosing a stamped addressed envelope is helpful if you write to any of the following organisations.

Adhesions Helpline *Tel:* 0345 023746 Information about adhesions and their prevention is available on this Helpline.

Amarant Centre 80 Lambeth Road, London SE1 7PW *Tel:* (020) 7401 3855 *Fax:* (020) 7928 9134 *Helpline:* 01293 413000
The Centre aims to promote a better understanding of the menopause. It distributes information packs, videos and cassettes.

APROP (Action for the Proper Regulation of Private Hospitals) PO Box 418, Weybridge, Surrey KT13 OSJ
A pressure group formed by disaffected private hospital patients that is campaigning for government regulation of the independent healthcare sector.

AVMA *(Action for Victims of Medical Accidents)* 44 High Street, Croydon, Surrey CRO 1YB *Tel:* (020) 8686 8333 *Fax:* (020) 8667 9065
This is the only national organisation dealing specifically with medical accidents. It will help to assess what has happened, advise on what can be done and how to do it.

BACUP *(British Association of Cancer United Patients and their families and friends)* 3 Bath Place, Rivington Street, London EC2A 3DR *Tel:* (020) 7696 9003 *Freephone:* 0808 800 1234 *Fax:* (020) 7696 9002 *e-mail:* info@cancerbacup.org *Website:* www.cancerbacup.org
Information and supportive counselling service.

British Acupuncture Council 163 Jeddo Road, London W12 9HQ *Tel:* (020) 8735 0400 *Fax:* (020) 8735 0404 *e-mail:* info@acupuncture.org.uk *Website:* www.acupuncture.org.uk

The Council represents 1,800 acupuncturists offering patients an holistic approach to maintaining health and managing illness.

British Association for Counselling 37a Sheep Street, Rugby CV21 3BX *Tel:* 01788 578328
Information on counselling services.

British Complementary Medicine Association Kensington House, Imperial Square, Cheltenham, Gloucestershire GL50 1QZ *Tel:* 01242 519911 *Fax:* 01242 227765 *e-mail:* info@bcma.co.uk *Website:* www.bcma.co.uk
Practitioners registered with the BCMA through their professional organisations are bound by the Code of Conduct. Information about therapies and where they can be obtained is available from the BCMA.

British Homoeopathic Association Enterprises Ltd 27a Devonshire Street, London W1N 1RJ
Tel: (020) 7935 2163 *Website:* www.nhsconfed.net/bha
There are over 600 doctors in the Register of the Faculty of Homoeopathy and treatment is available from GPs in the NHS as well as clinics at hospitals in London, Glasgow, Liverpool, Bristol and Tunbridge Wells.

British Medical Acupuncture Society Newton House, Newton Lane, Whitley, Warrington, Cheshire WA4 4JA *Tel:* 01925 730727 *Fax:* 01925 730492 *e-mail:* Bmasadmin@aol.com *Website:* www. medical-acupuncture.co.uk
Formed in 1980 as an association of medical practitioners interested in acupuncture, its 1,700 members use acupuncture in hospitals or general practice.

Family Health Services Authorities have replaced the Family Practitioner Committees, and information about them can be obtained from the local District Health Authority, Public Libraries and the Post Office.

Foster's Bakery (Linda Kearns cake), Barnsley, Yorkshire *Tel:* 01226 381712
A cake containing plant oestrogens.

General Medical Council 178–202 Great Portland Street, London W1N 6JE *Tel:* (020) 7580 7642 *Fax:* (020) 7915 3641 *Website:* www. gmc-uk.org
The GMC can only investigate complaints which amount to serious

professional misconduct. This may include clinical matters but will primarily include complaints about the behaviour of a doctor.

Health Service Ombudsman for England Millbank Tower, Millbank, London SW1P 4QP *Tel:* (020) 7217 4051
The Ombudsman investigates complaints about the National Health Service (NHS) and complaints should be made within one year of the incident.

Hysterectomy Information and Support

**Elizabeth Banks (Basingstoke) *Tel:* 01256 357879

**Tricia Crisp (Basingstoke) *Tel:* 01256 850514

Helen Jackson (Swindon) *Tel:* 01793 338885 Helen also runs **Gynae C** *Website:* www.gynae-c.ndo.co.uk (A support group for women with gynaecological cancer.)

Jan (Bristol) *Tel:* 0117 9681767

Kelly (Swindon) *Tel:* 01793 532442

**Pat Nelson, 2 Mourne Close, Buckskin 2, Basingstoke, Hants RG22 5BD *Tel:* 01256 357879 *Website:* www.hants.gov.uk

Linda Newall, The Hysterectomy Association, Aynsley House, Chester Gardens, Church Gresley, Swadlincote, Derbyshire DE11 9PU. *Website:* www.hysterectomy-association.org.uk/index.htm

**Lee Puddick (Basingstoke) *Tel:* 01256 323077

Carol Wetherell, Ardeer, Rafford, Forres, Morayshire, Scotland IV36 ORU *Tel:* 01309 673178

Eileen Wilford (Leicester) *Tel:* 0116 2743529

**Members of the Hysterectomy, HRT and Menopause Support Group

The IBS Network Northern General Hospital, Sheffield S5 7AU *Tel:* 0114 2611531 (Ansaphone) *e-mail:* p.j.nunn@sheffield.ac.uk *Website:* www.uel.ac.uk/pers/C.P.Dancey/ibs.html
An independent self-help organisation for people with Irritable Bowel Syndrome.

The National Endometriosis Society 50 Westminster Palace Gardens, Artillery Row, London SW1P 1RL *Tel:* (020) 7222

2781 *Fax:* (020) 7222 2786 *Helpline:* (020) 7222 2776 *e-mail:* endoinfo@compuserve.com *Website:* www.endo.org.uk
Support and self-help for endometriosis sufferers.

National Institute of Medical Herbalists 56 Longbrook Street, Exeter, Devon EX4 6AH *Tel:* 01392 426022 *Fax:* 01392 498963 *e-mail:* nimh@ukexeter.freeserve.co.uk *Website:* www.btinternet.com/~nimh
All members carry the letters of their qualification after their name – MNIMH or FNIMH – and the Institute Secretary will send a register of practitioners.

The National Osteoporosis Society PO Box 10, Radstock, Bath BA3 3YB *Tel:* 01761 432472 *Fax:* 01761 471104 *Helpline:* 01761 431594
Information and booklets available, as well as a VHS video covering all aspects of osteoporosis.

National Relate Herbert Gray College, Little Church Street, Rugby CV21 3AP *Tel:* 01788 573241 *Fax:* 01788 535007 *Website:* www.relate.org.uk
Counselling for couples or individuals with problems in their relationships.

N Films 78 Holyhead Road, Handsworth, Birmingham B21 OLH *Tel:* 0121 507 0341 A video about hysterectomy in English, Hindi, Urdu, Punjabi, Gujerati and Bengali is available for sale or hire.

Ovacome St Bartholomew's Hospital, West Smithfield, London EC1A 7BE. *Tel:* 07071 781861 *e-mail:* ovacome@ovacome.org.uk *Website:* www.ovacome.org.uk
Ovacome is a nationwide support group for all those concerned with ovarian cancer – sufferers, families, friends, carers and health professionals.

The SHE Trust Red Hall Lodge Offices, Red Hall Drive, Bracebridge Heath, Lincoln LN4 2JT *Tel/Fax:* 01522 519992
The Trust aims to promote awareness of endometriosis amongst the public, and has embarked on the first ever research into the on-going progress of endometriosis sufferers.

The Society of Homoeopaths 2 Artizan Road, Northampton NN1 4HU *Tel:* 01604 621400 *Fax:* 01604 622622 *e-mail:*

Societyofhomoeopaths@btinternet.com *Websites:* www.homoeopathy.
org.uk *and* www.hom-inform.org
The Society will put you in touch with a private homoeopathic
practitioner.

Women's Health 52–54 Featherstone Street, London EC1Y 8RT
Tel: (020) 7251 6580 *e-mail:* womenshealth@pop3.poptel.org.uk
A national information centre with large resource library, it publishes
a newsletter and puts women in touch with healthcare organisations
throughout the country.

Women's Nutritional Advisory Service PO Box 268, Lewes, East
Sussex BN7 2QN *Tel:* 01273 487366 *email:* wnas@wnas.org.uk
website: http://www.wnas.org.uk
The service provides help and information on treating women's
health problems by nutritional means. It specialises in PMS, IBS and
natural HRT.

*The first edition of my book (Virago, 1993) is available on cassette
and in braille for women who are blind or partially-sighted from:*
Customer Services, Royal National Institute for the Blind, RNIB
Peterborough, PO Box 173, Peterborough PE2 6WS *Tel:* 0345 023
153 *Fax:* 01733 371555 *e-mail:* cservices@rnib.org.uk

Selected Bibliography

Aberdeen Endometrial Ablation Trials Group. A randomised trial of endometrial ablation versus hysterectomy for the treatment of dysfunctional uterine bleeding: outcome at four years. *Br J Obstet Gynaecol* 1999; 106: 360–366

Amso, N.N., Stabinsky S.A., McFaul P., Blanc B., Pendley L., Neuwirth R., 'Uterine thermal balloon therapy for the treatment of menorrhagia: the first 300 patients from a multi-centre study'. *Br J Obstet Gynaecol* 1998; 105: 517–24

Belchetz, P., 'Hormone Replacement Therapy', *British Medical Journal*, Vol. 298, June 1989

Booth, M., Beral, V. and Smith, P., 'Risk Factors for Ovarian Cancer: a Case Control Study', *British Journal Cancer*, 60, May 1989

Bradley, E.A., Reidy, J.F., Forman, R.G., Jarosz, J., Braude, P.R., 'Transcatheter uterine artery embolisation to treat large uterine fibroids'. *Br J Obstet Gynaecol* 1998; 105: 235–40

Broome, A. and Wallace, L., *Psychology and Gynaecological Problems*, Tavistock Publications, London, 1984

Brunton, N., *Homoeopathy*, Optima, 1989

Campbell, Dr A., *Natural Health Handbook*, Apple Press, 1984

Celso-Ramon Garcia, Berg Cutler Winnifred, 'Preservation of the ovary: a re-evaluation'. *Fertility and Sterility* The American Fertility Society. Vol 42, No 4, October 1984

Coleman, Dr V., *Guide to Alternative Medicine*, Corgi Books, 1988

Coltart, T. and Smart, F., *The Woman's Guide to Surgery*, Thorsons, 1992

Coope, Dr J., *The Menopause: Coping with the Change*, Optima, 1988

Cooper, W., *No Change*, Arrow Books, 1976

Coppen, A. and Bishop, M., 'Hysterectomy, Hormones and Behaviour', *The Lancet*, January 1981.

Coulter, A. et al., 'Do British Women Undergo Too Few or Too Many Hysterectomies?' *Social Science Medicine*, Vol 27, No 9, 1988

Davis, H. and Fallowfield, L., *Counselling and Communication in Health Care*, Wiley, 1991

DeCherney, A. and Polan, M., 'Hysteroscopic Management of Intrauterine Lesions and Intractable Uterine Bleeding', *Obstetrics and Gynecology*, Vol 61, No 3, March 1983

DeCherney, A. et al., 'Endometrial Ablation for Intractable Uterine Bleeding: Hysteroscopic Resection', *Obstetrics and Gynecology*, Vol 70, No 4, October 1987

Firebrace, P. and Hill, S., *New Ways to Health. A Guide to Acupuncture*, Hamlyn, 1988

Fish, S., 'Hormone Replacement Therapy', *Nursing Mirror*, August 1983

Goodwin, S.C., Vedanthum, S., McLucas, B., Forno, A.E., Parellà, R., 'Preliminary experience with uterine artery embolisation for uterine fibroids'. *J Vasc Intervent Radiol* 1997; 8: 517–26

Gould, D., 'Hidden Problems after Hysterectomy', *Nursing Times*, June 1986

Green, A. et al. 'Tubal sterilisation, hysterectomy and decreased risk of ovarian cancer'. *Int J Cancer* 1997; 71: 948–951

Guy's Hospital Reports, Vol 78, 1928 (available on order from local libraries)

Guyton, A.C., *Textbook of Medical Physiology*, Saunders, 1966

Harvey, J. et al., *Cervical Cancer and How to Stop Worrying About It*, Faber and Faber, 1988

Haslett, S., 'Hysterectomy Counselling', *Nursing Mirror*, Vol 161, No 16, October 1985

Hayman, S., *Endometriosis*, Penguin Books, 1991

Hoffman, D., *The Holistic Herbal*, Element Books, 1983

Hufnagel, V., *No More Hysterectomies*, Thorsons, 1990

Hutchins Jr. F.L., Worthington-Kirsch, R., Berkowitz, R.P., 'Selective Uterine Artery Embolisation as Primary Treatment for Symptomatic Leiomyomata Uteri', *The Journal of the American Association of Gynecologic Laparascopists*. August 1999, Vol 6, No 3

Jackson, B.B., *Role of Social Resource Variables upon Life Satisfaction in Black Climacteric Hysterectomised Women*, School of Nursing, McGill University, Quebec, Nursing Papers, 1985

Jordan, J., *Light-Knives in Gynaecology*, World Medicine, July 1984

Junor, P., *What Every Woman Needs to Know*, Century, 1988

Key, E., 'Advances in Hormone Replacement Therapy', *Nursing Standard*, July 1991

Kitzinger, S., *Woman's Experience of Sex*, Penguin Books, 1983

Lehrer S., 'Tubal litigation, hysterectomy, and risk of ovarian cancer', *JAMA* 1994 Apr 27; 271 (16): 1236

Le Strange, R., *A History of Herbal Plants*, Angus and Robertson, 1977

Lincoln, Prof. D.W., 'The Human Uterus in Health, Redundancy and Distress, *MRC News*, March 1988

Loft, A., et al., 'Incidence of ovarian cancer after hysterectomy: a nationwide controlled follow up', *Br J Obstet Gynaecol* 1997 Nov; 104 (11) 1296–301

Magos, A., et al., 'Transcervical Resection of Endometrium in Women with Menorrhagia', *British Medical Journal*, Vol 298, May 1989

Mann, F., *Scientific Aspects of Acupuncture*, Heinemann, 1977

Mayes, K., *Brittle Bones and the Calcium Crisis*, Grapevine, 1987

McLucas, B., Goodwin, S., Vedanthum, S., 'Embolic therapy for myomata', *Minimally Invasive & Allied Technology* 1996; 5: 336–338

Melville, A., *Natural Hormone Health*, Thorsons, 1990

Mersey Regional Drug Information Service, Drug Information Letter *Hormone Replacement Therapy*, July 1991

Mills, S., *Out of the Earth: the Essential Book of Herbal Medicine*, Viking, 1991

O'Connor, H., Broadbent, J.A., Magos, A.L., McPherson, K., 'Medical Research Council randomised trial of endometrial resection versus hysterectomy in management of menorrhagia', *Lancet* 1997; 349: 887–901

O'Connor, H., Magos, A., 'Endometrial resection for the treatment of menorrhagia', *N Engl J Med* 1995; 335: 151–6

Overton, C., Hargreaves, J., Maresh. M., 'A national survey of the complications of endometrial resection for menstrual disorders: the MISTLETOE study', *Br J Obstet Gynaecol* 1997; 104: 1351–9

Paskowitz, R.A. ' "Rollerball" ablation of the endometrium', *J Reprod Med* 1995; 40: 333–6

Payer, L., *Medicine Culture*, Gollancz, 1989

Pearson, P., *Acupuncture*, MTP Press, 1987

Philipp, Dr E., *Hysterectomy*, British Medical Association, 1987

Povov, A., 'Homoeopathy in Treatment of Patients with Fibromyoma of the Uterus', *British Homoeopathic Journal*, 1992

Ravina, J.H. et. al., 'Arterial embolisation to treat uterine myomata', *The Lancet* 1995; Vol 346: 671–672

Rees, M., 'Modern Management of Menorrhagia', *Hospital Update*, May 1992

Richardson, S., *New Ways to Health. A Guide to Homoeopathy*, Hamlyn, 1988

Royal College of Obstetricians and Gynaecologists. Report of the RCOG working party on training in gynaecological endoscopic surgery (June 1994), London, RCOG Press

Schairer, C. et al., 'Estrogen-Progesten Hormone Replacement Therapy associated with greater increase in breast cancer risk than therapy with estrogen alone', JAMA 2000; 283: 485–491

Scottish Medicines Resource Centre, *Hormone Replacement Therapy and the Menopause*, December 1991

Sharp, N.C., Cronin, N., Feldberg, I., Evans, N., Hodgson, D., Ellis, S., 'Microwaves for menorrhagia: a new fast technique for endometrial ablation', *Lancet* 1995; 346: 1003–1004

Shorter, E., *Doctors and their Patients*, Transaction, 1991

Siddle, N., Sarrel, P., Whitehead, M., 'The effect of hysterectomy on the age at ovarian failure: identification of a subgroup of women with premature loss of ovarian function', *Fertility & Sterility* Vol.47, No 1, January 1987

South Western Regional Drug Information Centre, 'Prescribing Points', *Hormone Replacement Therapy*, March 1992

Survey of Women's Health Study Group, 'Tubal sterilisation, hysterectomy and decreased risk of ovarian cancer', *Int J Cancer* 1997 Jun 11; 71(6): 948–951

Wangcheng, L. et al., 'Acupuncture Treatment of Functional Uterine Bleeding – a clinical observation of 30 cases', *Journal of Traditional Chinese Medicine*, Vol. 8, No. 1, 1988

Webb, C. and Wilson-Barnett, J., 'Hysterectomy: Dispelling the Myths – 1', *Nursing Times*, November 1983

Wheeler, C., *An Introduction to the Principles and Practice of Homoeopathy*, Eastern Press, 1982

Which? *Complementary Medicine*, 1986.

Wilks, S. and Bettany, G., *Biographical History of Guy's Hospital*, Ward Lock and Brown, 1892.

Wright, S., 'Conspiracy of Silence', *Nursing Mirror*, May 1985

Yaegashi, N., et. al., 'Incidence of ovarian cancer in women with prior hysterectomy in Japan', *Gynaecol Oncol*. 1998 Mar; 68(3): 244–6

Zussman, L. et al., 'Sexual Response after Hysterectomy-Oophorectomy: Recent Studies and Reconsideration of Psychogenesis', *American Journal of Obstetrics and Gynecology*, Vol.140, No.7, August 1981

Index